Agency and Bodily Autonomy in Systems of Care

ANTHROPOLOGY OF WELL-BEING

Individual, Community, Society

Series Editor

Mary Cameron, Florida Atlantic University

Mission Statement

Well-being is central and important in people's daily lives and life history. This book series brings about understanding of what the complex concepts of well-being include. The concepts of quality of life, life satisfaction, and happiness will be explored and viewed at the individual level, the community level, and the level of society. The series encourages and promotes research into the concept of well-being, how it appears to be defined culturally, and how it is utilized across levels and across different social, economic, and ethnic groups. Understandings of how well-being promotes stability and resilience will also be critical to advances in understanding, as well as how well-being can be implemented as a goal in resisting vulnerabilities and in adaptation. Series books include monographs and edited collections by a range of academics, from rising scholars to experts in relevant fields.

Recent Titles in the Series

Agency and Bodily Autonomy in Systems of Care, edited by Heidi M. Altman
Drug Use, Recovery, and Maternal Instinct Bias: A Biocultural and Social-Ecological Approach, by Caitlyn D. Placek
Entanglements of Rare Diseases in the Baltic Sea Region, edited by Małgorzata Rajtar and Katarzyna E. Król
The Moral Evaluation of Emergency Department Patients: An Ethnography of Triage Work in Romania, by Marius Wamsiedel
Well-Being as a Multidimensional Concept: Understanding Connections among Culture, Community, and Health, edited by Janet M. Page-Reeves
Boundaries of Care: Community Health Workers in the United States, by Ryan I. Logan
Clinical Anthropology 2.0: Improving Medical Education and Patient Experience, edited by Jason W. Wilson and Roberta D. Baer
Living with HIV in Post-Crisis Times: Beyond the Endgame, edited by David A. B. Murray

Agency and Bodily Autonomy in Systems of Care

Edited by Heidi M. Altman

LEXINGTON BOOKS
Lanham • Boulder • New York • London

Published by Lexington Books
An imprint of The Rowman & Littlefield Publishing Group, Inc.
4501 Forbes Boulevard, Suite 200, Lanham, Maryland 20706
www.rowman.com

86-90 Paul Street, London EC2A 4NE

British Library Cataloguing in Publication Information Available

Library of Congress Cataloging-in-Publication Data

Names: Altman, Heidi M., 1965- editor.
Title: Agency and bodily autonomy in systems of care / edited by Heidi M. Altman.
Description: Lanham : Lexington Books, [2024]. | Series: Anthropology of well-being: individual, community, society | Includes bibliographical references and index. | Summary: "Agency and Bodily Autonomy in Systems of Care examines how humans and their bodies become enmeshed in systems of care. This book establishes the need for advocacy and policy change to improve health outcomes by re-envisioning systems of care as spaces that include individual agency and bodily autonomy"-- Provided by publisher.
Identifiers: LCCN 2023053293 (print) | LCCN 2023053294 (ebook) | ISBN 9781666952704 (cloth) | ISBN 9781666952728 (paperback) | ISBN 9781666952711 (epub)
Subjects: LCSH: Medical personnel and patient--Case studies. | Patient-centered health care--Case studies. | Social medicine--Case studies. | Right to bodily autonomy--Case studies. | Human body--Social aspects--Case studies.
Classification: LCC R727.3 .A355 2024 (print) | LCC R727.3 (ebook) | DDC 610.69/6--dc23/eng/20240112
LC record available at https://lccn.loc.gov/2023053293
LC ebook record available at https://lccn.loc.gov/2023053294

I would like to express my gratitude to Kristin D. Meeuwen, who served as my editorial assistant in the production of this volume.

Contents

Preface

The work in this volume began as a conversation in the spring of 2022, while several of the authors were at Georgia Southern University for a presentation by Cindi SturtzSreetharan. Her recent work on the volume *Fat in Four Cultures* made for a fascinating public lecture and during our time together we began to think about the ways in which our work intersected, connecting linguistic, cultural, and applied anthropology as well as public health. We became fascinated by the similarities of the experiences of the people we worked with, even though it would seem that we have disparate fields of interest. The unifying connection was the human body vs. the various institutions that would try, and often succeed, to control it.

As we parted ways, we agreed to organize a session at that year's American Anthropological Association meeting in Seattle to take up the themes that we had in common. That session included presentations from Altman, Berger, Smallwood, SturtzSreetharan, and Sweeney Tookes. During the session, and in discussion with members of the audience, we were gratified to see that the connections we had proposed in our conversations were relevant when supported by data from fieldwork, collections research and government data.

Seeing the potential for further collaboration we recruited two more authors with connections to the overall theme, Odusanya and White, and began the process of constructing this volume. As we did so, it became clear that the connections between our work run deep in reflecting theories of how bodies are controlled or managed, but especially how this happens in the context of medical institutions. Whether we use the lenses of Foucault or Bourdieu or Butler or approach our work from an applied or advocacy perspective, common themes emerge. Our bodies are the places where all elements of culture and society converge. We have limited agency in determining our health outcomes when we interact with systems of care. In the work presented here, this limited agency has negative effects on our health outcomes, whether they be damage or injury to our physical body or lasting impact on our psychological and emotional health. Given these findings, our work also emerges as set of evidence-based pleas for advocacy on behalf of anyone entering into a system of care.

Acknowledgments

CHAPTER 3

Generous support for this research was provided by the Abe Fellowship/ Social Science Research Council.

CHAPTER 5

The interviews analyzed for this chapter were conducted during several different projects, and we would like to thank the funders who made this research possible: Georgia Department of Natural Resources Coastal Resource Division, University of Georgia Marine Extension and Georgia Sea Grant, and the National Marine Fisheries Service's Marine Fisheries Initiative.

We would also like to express gratitude to the Georgia Southern University Anthropology students who assisted with data collection, and most importantly, the patient and generous people of the fishing communities of Georgia and South Carolina.

CHAPTER 7

Abiding gratitude to the Georgia Southern University College of Behavioral and Social Sciences, Office of Research Support and Sponsored Programs (and the Provost's Office), and the Department of Sociology and Anthropology for support of this project. The College provided seed money that paid for crucial student assistance as I was beginning to process the data for this project. The Research Office and Provost's Office provided funding through the Research Impact Accelerator program to fund my summer work and a graduate assistant. The department and my colleagues awarded me educational leave to move this project along. Without this support I could not have continued this labor of love.

Special thanks, also, to the student volunteers and paid assistants who have helped with the data cleaning, coding and analysis on this project including, especially, Alexis McGhee.

Finally, an enduring debt of appreciation and gratitude for the community partners and agencies who support and facilitate this work without fail, especially Dr. Nkenge Jackson, the Willow Hill Heritage and Renaissance Center, the Curtis V. Cooper Clinics, the Medical College of Georgia, and Restoring the Breach.

Introduction

Heidi M. Altman

When we enter into any system that regulates our bodies, whether it be a penal system, a military system, or systems designed to manage health, prevent illness, repair injury, or even to administer insurance for our bodies, we lose control of some of the most fundamental aspects of who we are as human beings—our sense of agency and our ability to determine what happens to ourselves. Even in situations in which we have the right or the ability to negotiate our experience within complex systems, we rarely have the autonomy to make all the decisions for ourselves, and in many instances, we would prefer not to have to make those decisions. We as individuals often do not know, for example, the best course of treatment for complex illnesses or the best means for achieving particular goals with regard to our health. In industrialized nations like the United States, we train and engage medical specialists who are charged with knowing the minutiae of each bodily system, although this sometimes results in losing sight of treating the whole person.

The intersections of gender, age, ability, ethnicity, class, race, and language also impact our positions as agents in our own care in ways that can influence health outcomes. The loss of agency at these critical moments is the central theme of this volume. How do individuals in the contemporary world make room for themselves in healthcare situations? Our humanness lies in a negotiation between our bodies, our culture and the society that would control us. The papers in this volume explore this complex negotiation as it exists for bodies that are inherently subject to a system of care outside the control of the person who inhabits them. The fieldwork sites in these chapters vary from Italy, to Japan, to the American South, but each features questions that focus our understanding of culture, embodiment and agency on the individual who is being subjected to systems of "care," which can also be understood as systems of control. Controlling the bodies of individuals by medical treatment (or the lack thereof) is a central concern of these papers.

How the body exists as a location for establishing, performing and negotiating agency and autonomy is a long-standing question within philosophy, and within social and cultural anthropology for at least one hundred years. While what follows is by no means an exhaustive catalogue of philosophical and anthropological positions on the body and experiences of agency and autonomy, it is meant to highlight the paradigms that are relevant to the chapters presented here. With the development of the postmodern movement in the social sciences, the notion of bodily autonomy emerged as a question of lived experience versus inscription; of the body as a representational object of study or the experiences of the body as phenomenology. Refinements of this question that take culture, position, and performance into consideration have become a central concern of medical anthropology, cultural anthropology and even linguistic anthropology. A review of the relevant literature provides context for the chapters in this volume, and outlining questions of gender, sexuality, ability/disability, consent, and autonomy are particularly relevant.

THEORETICAL FOUNDATIONS

In the early part of the twentieth century social theorists were developing the models for the structures of society and culture that are foundational to our understanding today. In his 1935 essay "Techniques of the Body" Marcel Mauss, French sociologist and anthropologist (one of the first to postulate the role of society and culture in the development of human bodies across the life span), enumerates the ways in which virtually all of the ways the body can be moved or used are shaped by the culture in which the individual is immersed. This enumeration resulted from Mauss's realization that culturally significant information about the body and its techniques was being relegated to the category of "miscellaneous" in the ethnology of the day. In order afford cultural significance to the body, Mauss described these "techniques" as learned behaviors that begin with imitation of prestigious individuals, but through repetition and the enforcement of the techniques by the process of education and the authority of the prestigious individuals, these techniques become reflections of cultural norms. These include ways of walking, swimming, dancing, climbing, having sex, giving birth, etc. Each potential realm of physical activity has a cultural component, even explicitly biological functions, like excretion. He asserts that the techniques he describes must be "effective and traditional. There is no technique and no transmission in the absence of tradition. This above all is what distinguishes man from the animals: the transmission of his techniques and very probably their oral transmission" (1935, 75). Thus, Mauss launches social theory into an examination of the body as a subject for understanding cultural patterns and the relationships between biology/physiology, sociology/anthropology, and psychology.

While Mauss lay the foundations for examining and interpreting the ways in which physical behaviors are shaped through cultural transmission, his observations and formulations were more specifically focused on social and cultural institutions rather than on the body itself. Mauss sets forth lists of areas for investigation including how the techniques could be classified, the ways in which the techniques vary across the life span and the sexes, and potential domains for investigation. As anthropology continued to develop into a field of its own, firsthand observations and participant observation became the hallmark of the field, and the observational data collected by trained anthropologists enlarged the basis for ethnological comparisons of various bodily habits or techniques.

The description of the body, and the cultural practices that shape it, takes an outsider's perspective in the work of Mauss and other early anthropologists. Understanding culture from the perspective of insiders began to emerge in anthropology in the early to mid twentieth century as extended seasons of fieldwork led participant observers to begin to feel as though they were part of the communities they studied. Meanwhile, Maurice Merleau-Ponty, a French philosopher at the middle of the twentieth century, built upon the German philosophical tradition of phenomenology and focused on the ways in which the body is a locus for feeling and experience. In his seminal work *Phenomenology of Perception* (1945), Merleau-Ponty asserts that the body is not an object for medicine to encounter, nor is it simply a home for our consciousness. Rather, the body is the self, the means for both experience and consciousness of experience. In terms of the development of philosophy, this was a radical notion, because Merleau-Ponty posits that bodily experiences are recognizable as feelings before the reflection of consciousness. This point of view intersected with the development of existentialism and his fundamental claim that the experiences, time and space of the body itself were essential to consciousness provided fertile ground for the development of existentialism. For the purposes of this volume and our various considerations of the body, Merleau-Ponty's revolutionary ideas about the phenomenology of the body in the world are most important. Several of the chapters include firsthand narratives of medical experiences that reflect individuals' time in systems of care. These narratives, in part, allow us observe that individuals are conscious of their body's knowledge, even when confronted with systems that seek to control the discourse around their experience.

Contrary to Merleau-Ponty's phenomenology, Michel Foucault understood the human experience through other lenses, notably the unconscious structure models asserted by the French structuralists, including Claude Levi-Strauss. Foucault's classic work *Discipline and Punish: The Birth of the Prison* (1977) continues his depiction of the human body as an element under the control of outside structures, whether they be carceral, military or medical. In the medical context, according to Foucault there are

> two correlative possibilities: firstly, the constitution of the individual as a describable analyzable object not in order to reduce him to "specific" features, as did the naturalists in relation to living beings, but in order to maintain him in his individual features, in his particular evolution, in his own aptitudes or abilities, under the gaze of a permanent corpus of knowledge; and, secondly, the constitution of a comparative system that made possible the measurement of overall phenomena, the description of groups, the characterization of collective facts, the calculation of the gaps between individuals, their distribution in a given "population." (190)

In other words, Foucault shows that the development of the system of medical observation and record-keeping establishes the human body both as an object unto itself and as a representation of a group, foundational to his idea of biopower. Foucault's work shows that the development of modern medicine allowed for a consolidation of medical authority and the concomitant objectification of human experience, a construction of the body far from the phenomenology of Merleau-Ponty. For Foucault, the act of description, the use of language to label and define, provides medical practitioners a discourse of their own about the body that excludes the patient from being an interlocutor and thereby reduces their illness or disease to symptoms or pathologies that the practitioner can observe. However, the authority possessed by the practitioner inscribes their observation on the body of the patient, who, without authority or access to medical discourse, is thereby controlled. For the authors in this volume, the questions and paradigms established by Foucault are central to aspects of our understanding of medical anthropology and figure significantly into our examinations of particular cases in which individuals and groups interact with medical spaces. In these chapters, agency, autonomy, consent and exclusion from medical discourse figure prominently.

Bourdieu, a contemporary of Foucault, considered the body as well, however, for him the body was a reflection of and embodiment of the social structures that surrounded it, with power and authority being cast as mechanisms of social and cultural capital. In *Outline of a Theory of Practice* (1977), Bourdieu uses ethnographic examples of rites and rituals to demonstrate his assertions that the habitus is the way in which the body is shaped by cultural factors, and that the internalized cultural factors are the way in which it knows how to interact with the world. In this paradigm, an individual's cultural capital is expressed through aspects of the body that have significance in the culture. At the same time, the body is the location of the embodiment of social and cultural beliefs and practices known as the habitus, as well as the place where aspects of symbolic capital are expressed (the embodied habitus is labelled the hexis). Bourdieu strikes a middle path between the strictly experiential phenomenology of Merleau-Ponty and the structural examination of power structures vis-à-vis the body asserted by Foucault. For Bourdieu,

> Body hexis speaks directly to the motor function, in the form of a pattern of postures that is both individual and systematic, because linked to a whole system of techniques involving the body and tools, and charged with a host of social meanings and values: in all societies, children are particularly attentive to the gestures and postures which, in their eyes, express everything that goes to make an accomplished adult. (87)

In Bourdieu's model, the culture is embodied through mimesis or in a larger sense by practice. Practice drawn broadly includes all of the rites and experiences one employs in the development of the habitus and in the accumulation and engagement of cultural capital. These take shape in seen and unseen aspects of the body. Where Foucault sees the body as the locus of power struggles, through regulation, management, and control by authorities, Bourdieu sees the body as the product and reflection of social structures and power systems. For Bourdieu, the body itself is a form of cultural capital with prestige afforded to those who embody cultural preferences, and those who conform their bodies in that way. This theme is reflected these chapters, especially in discussions of stigma, self-criticism and policing the body.

Judith Butler, a philosopher of gender, builds on the work of Foucault and Bourdieu to contend that individuals enact and embody gender roles through everyday actions (1990). Her assertion that gender is performative indicates that gender as we recognize it relies on the repetition of gendered behaviors that are consistent with societal norms. When individuals consistently perform these behaviors, they contribute to the stabilization of gender categories. Performativity also leaves ample room for individuals to challenge societal norms through their actions and thereby can destabilize and redefine socially recognized gender categories. There is pressure from society to conform, but also agency within individuals to rebel and create change. In other words, for Butler, performativity is "the process by which discourse produces the effects that it names" (Butler 1990, 145). Although not strictly anthropological, Butler's work has had far-reaching impact in many fields that use it as a theoretical base. Feminist scholars use Butler's paradigm to analyze how gender roles are constructed and disrupted. Intersectional theorists have built upon Butler's ideas to explore how various aspects of identity, including gender, race, class, and sexuality, intersect and influence each other. The concept of performativity can be applied to understand how individuals navigate and perform multiple identities in different social contexts. In anthropology this model is foundational to our understanding of embodiment being more than just the experience of phenomena. The body is a locus for stabilizing norms and expectations, but also for subverting them by upending our cultural assumptions about the association between sex and gender.

Turning now to the theoretical and methodological practices of anthropology, specifically, we see that at approximately the same time as Foucault and Bourdieu's work was gaining traction, anthropologist Clifford Geertz, and other symbolic anthropologists, were developing the symbolic/interpretive paradigm. Geertz's model of symbolic anthropology advocates for what he calls "thick description" to capture all elements of the cultural context, and then interpreting the described event through the community's lens. The method prescribed by Geertz is designed to allow ethnographers (and readers) to interpret cultural events and practices as an insider would (1972). The subjectivity of this method aligns closely with the phenomenological approaches to culture and experience outlined by Merleau-Ponty. Geertz asserts that this method is not simply the physical experience, but the interpretation that situates a given experience or action within its complete cultural context. Geertz and the symbolic anthropologists found themselves at odds with materialists (like Marvin Harris), however the subjective methods promulgated by Geertz had a lasting impact on ethnographers and the methods of ethnography.

As an example of the persistence of thick description as a method in the interpretation of cultures, the work of Scheper-Hughes continues this practice, but she turns her gaze toward the cultural constructions of motherhood, the various forms of violence against the body and even the trafficking in human organs. While she is an ethnographer, she is also a former nurse and medical anthropologist who is concerned with the body and its treatment in many contexts. In *Death Without Weeping* (1993) Scheper-Hughes describes herself as being "engaged here in an ongoing work of praxis—theory derived in the context of political practice" (170). In her work we see not just the work of the ethnographer, but that of an advocate whose political action is derived from the deep observational experiences of ethnography. However, she takes anthropology to task for being complicit in the power structures that perpetuate individuals participating in their own inequality. She says, "as social scientists (not social revolutionaries) critical practice implies for us not so much a practical as an epistemological struggle. Here the contested domain is anthropology itself. It concerns the way in which knowledge is generated, the interests it serves, and the challenge to make our discipline more relevant and nonoppressive to the people we study" (172). This call to action is echoed throughout her work in medical and applied anthropology and rings through the chapters presented here.

WORK IN THIS VOLUME

As one might imagine, because all the works in this volume discuss systems of care the works of Foucault feature prominently, but there are other paradigms that connect them as well. Berger's chapter explores the postmortem treatment and agency of historical patients using a structural violence framework and shows how understandings of past transgressions can inform current and future scholarship grounded in respect and dignity. Documentary and osteological analyses of the Siena Craniological Collection (SCC) from Siena, Italy, illustrate that there has been a general lack of care and respect for asylum patient remains postmortem, both in original skeletal preparation and subsequent management, storage, and use. By examining this process and its implications through the lens of structural violence, Berger presents a more complete picture regarding how lower-status, mentally ill individuals were transformed without their consent from community members to psychiatric patients, and finally, into objects of study as anatomical specimens. These novel findings also demonstrate the value of more detailed taphonomic data and how it can speak to questions of institutional patient agency, ethical anthropological research, and the construction of memory.

In a contemporary examination of disability, Odusanya's discussion of the autonomy and consent of children with intellectual and developmental disabilities and their parents is written through public health paradigms but recounts the history and complexity of disability studies from an advocacy perspective. She uses an intersectional lens to explore the recent designation of people with disabilities as a community with health disparities, which prompts the consideration of social determinants of health and the health outcomes they impact. Notions of stigma and agency feature in her discussion as well as Bourdieu's focus on the body as a locus and reflection of social capital. She shows that systemic oppression directed toward people with disabilities consists of numerous violations of body autonomy, including but not limited to being subjected to medical inspectors to determine whether a person with a disability was a public charge; sterilization to promote eugenics, institutionalization, and being used as objects for entertainment. Her particular focus on children and youth with special healthcare needs (CYSHCN) highlights the findings from interviews with parents of adolescents with Down syndrome (DS), in addition to the adolescents with DS themselves, pertaining to the dietary, physical activity, and social behaviors of adolescents with DS in South Georgia. Her findings underscore the lack of body autonomy for adolescents with DS at the individual level in addition to the lack of body autonomy at the interpersonal level in relation to the impact of parents/caregivers' decisions.

Foucault's notions of biopower and institutional control of individuals are readily apparent in SturtzSreetharan's examination of Japanese masculinity, government intervention, and body shaming. The Japanese government's proactive interventions to prevent obesity and metabolic disorder in the population take the form of annual checks of each individual's health through biometrics and diagnostic testing for people aged 40–74. Although the national rates for obesity are low, the stakes are high for individuals who experience the shame of not measuring up. She shows that men experience judgements that link large bodies to social failure, public shaming, and internalized stigma. In this context internalized vigilance of one's own body translated to anti-fat sentiment about oneself. Hypervigilance and self-blame are linked to perceptions of self-discipline and even morality.

The themes of masculinity and self-perception are central Sweeney Tookes and her coauthors' ethnographic work among commercial fishers in the US state of Georgia. The fishers, who are predominantly men, engage in a hazardous profession rife with work-related injuries, and nutrition and stress-related health conditions. They are also fiercely independent, and cope with the dangerous nature of their work through the use of external inputs to their bodies, and internal coping mechanisms to mediate the stress of this danger. Regardless, injuries and illnesses do occur, and fishers use these instances of pain and suffering to demonstrate their strong work ethic, to assert masculinity through their ability to work while injured, and to exercise agency and bodily autonomy via their refusal to seek medical treatment in an expedient manner. This chapter explores emic perspectives about illness and injury, particularly around healthcare-seeking behaviors.

Smallwood and Adom's examination of queer bodies and the stigma of PrEP use focuses our attention on stigmatized identities from a public health perspective. The Centers for Disease Control report that there are currently approximately 1.2 million people living with HIV in the United States, with approximately 37,000 new diagnoses in 2019, and pre-exposure prophylaxis (PrEP) has been identified as a highly successful biomedical intervention to reduce the risk of HIV infection from sex by more than 90 percent (Centers for Disease Control and Prevention, 2022). Smallwood and Adom show that although there is considerable empirical evidence for its efficacy, many individuals who are indicated for PrEP are not engaging in uptake. Reasons for refusing PrEP uptake include stigmas associated with PrEP use, such as perceptions of promiscuity and fear of judgment from healthcare providers (Calabrese, 2020; Brooks et al., 2019). This chapter focuses on the dynamics between informed decision making and the power structures that impose control on queer bodies. Smallwood and Adom use qualitative data to provide insight about the ways in which individual autonomy and sociocultural factors influence PrEP uptake.

White's partially autoethnographic account of breastfeeding considers the pressure to wean for people who breastfeed/chestfeed children for two years or more in the United States. This pressure takes many forms and comes from many sources. White explores the popular imaginaries about appropriate weaning times that have emerged after the widespread introduction of formula. She shows that many people who nurse children beyond infancy and toddlerhood are told that they are doing it "just for comfort." This chapter focuses specifically on the ways medical and legal professionals and institutions wield power to control and coerce caregivers to wean their children abruptly and before they are ready, often with negative emotional, psychological, and physical consequences. White demonstrates that biomedical professionals and the legal system chip away at the bodily autonomy of breastfeeding/chestfeeding parents and their children and diminish the agency that is often already constrained by pressure from family and work-related pressures to wean. Racial identity, income, education, gender identity, and other factors intersect in the social and cultural capital that parents/caregivers can draw on to resist these external threats to their parenting decisions.

Women in Georgia are at the intersection of social, political and economic forces that leave them with few opportunities for agency in Altman and Oloyede's exploration of maternity care, bodily autonomy, and control. This chapter demonstrates that when women enter into systems that do not take their agency, personhood and autonomy into consideration, negative health outcomes can result. In a state with one of the highest maternal mortality rates in the United States, the data collected in this chapter indicate that women experience their maternity care with a variety of responses, but a recurring theme in their narratives is that they feel out of control during pregnancy, labor/delivery, and the postpartum year. This chapter examines their narratives of (lack of) autonomy and how the culture of care in Georgia is structured to diminish their ability to feel in control of their bodies. Women in this study who experience diminished agency often experience adverse events during their maternity care. The critical role of agency in maternal health outcomes is highlighted through descriptions of dehumanization and the physical harm endured by women's pregnant bodies.

Throughout these chapters, we witness individuals who must submit (or refuse to submit) to medical institutions where their agency is curtailed or usurped. In each chapter, we can observe coercion or control creating a sense of dehumanization for people seeking care or being placed into systems of care against their wishes or without their knowledge. The stigmatization in these cases becomes internalized as self-blame and shame, which develops into an additional means of control for institutions to wield against those in need of care. Further, damage to the body features prominently in many of these accounts, pointing us again and again to the reality that structural violence has physical effects. Taken together, these chapters entreat us to advocacy for patient-centered care, for bodily autonomy, and for liberation from over-medicalization.

Chapter 1

Stewardship of Institutional and Historical Anatomical Skeletal Assemblages

A Case Study and Practical Recommendations

Jacqueline Berger

The year is 1862. You're a forty-year-old female in Siena, Italy. You've been admitted to the San Niccolò Psychiatric Hospital and diagnosed as an "imbecile." When you die, on a date that no one writes down, the examining doctor will note you died of a fever that seemed to "dissolve" you and that your frontal lobes appear to be atrophied. You are the first person anatomized for the hospital anatomical collection.

The year is 1865. You're a forty-three year-old male diagnosed with depression characterized by suicidal and homicidal tendencies. When you die on the 11th of August, still in the asylum, the examining doctor will note the asymmetry of your occipitals.

The year is 1904. You're a seventy-seven year-old female diagnosed with "consecutive" dementia. When you die on the 25th of July 1904, still in the asylum, they will simply note that you were murderous.

The year is 1931. You're a seventy-seven year-old male. When you die on the 3rd of January, the only note will be that you died in the asylum. Italy is changing and you will be the last of your kind—a person anatomized for the hospital anatomical collection.

Emblematic of a holistic vision of anthropology (Buikstra 2006; Zuckerman and Armelagos 2011), bioarchaeology has been defined as "the study of human remains from archaeological contexts, especially during the last 10,000 years of human evolution" (Larsen and Walker 2010, 380). Increasingly, "contexts" have come to include skeletal assemblages and their circumstances beyond the site from which the remains were recovered (Larsen and Walker 2010). The context of interest for this chapter is historical institutions and the skeletal assemblages often associated with them. Institutions are broadly defined as established and recognized organizations, especially those who provide care or assistance in some form, to a marginalized group such as the impoverished, disabled, or mentally ill (Baugher 2009). Institutions are often seen as exerting control over peoples' experiences, daily life, and autonomy. The study of these organizations using archaeological methods—institutional archaeology—began in the early to mid twentieth century with analyses of Spanish missions and their impact on Native American converts. The field has subsequently expanded to address communal societies: utopian communities; preindustrial institutions for the care of the poor, such as almshouses and workhouses; and nineteenth-century asylums—the latter often termed "total institutions" (Eghigian 2010; Shorter 1997). Earlier studies of these contexts have drawn upon remains of architecture, landscape design, and other artifacts as indications of institutional life and attitudes towards the marginalized; however, more recent studies have turned direct attention to the people of the past, apparent in the growth of a bioarchaeology focused on the life and death of institutionalized individuals (Baugher 2009; Berger 2021; Blakely 1997; Blakely and Harrington 1997a, 1997b; Collins 2009; Conlin Casella 2009; Crist, Mooney, and Morrell 2017; Curtis-Richardson 1997; De Cunzo 2009; DiGangi and Sirianni 2017; Fennelly 2014; Garcia-Putnam, Halling, and Seidemann 2023; Garcia-Putnam 2021; Geber 2015, 2016a, 2016b; Geber, Bergman, and Iregren 2019; Geber and Murphy 2012; Gibb 2009; Grauer and McNamara 1995; Halling and Seidemann 2017; Harrington and Blakely 1995; Higgins et al. 2002; Higgins and Sirianni 1995; Knowles and Sirianni 2014; Leavitt-Reynolds 2011; McGloin 2012; Muller 2017; Muller, Pearlstein, and de la Cova 2017; Murray and Perzigian 1995; Nystrom 2014, 2017a, 2017b; Nystrom et al. 2017; Phillips 2001, 2016; Piddock 2009; Sirianni and Higgins 1995; Sutter 1995), including the frequent collection of their remains in the furtherance of early anatomical study. This chapter explores one emblematic case study through a structural violence framework and addresses how bioarchaeologists can be more respectful and ethical stewards of institutional and historical anatomical skeletal assemblages. In the spirit of osteobiography (Boutin 2011, 2016; Boutin and Callahan 2019; Hawkey 1998; Robb 2002; Stodder and Palkovich 2012), this chapter began with small vignettes about various patients. This vision should serve as a guiding lens for the reader, namely, how can we personalize and humanize—via bioarchaeology—the lived experiences of the nineteenth- and early-twentieth-century asylum and use this to inform our research and stewardship?

CASE STUDY

Our case study focuses on one institution: *L'Ospedale Psichiatrico San Niccolò* or the San Niccolò Psychiatric Hospital, located in Siena, Italy. The San Niccolò was in operation from October 1818 until September 1999, serving patients in Siena, Italy and the surrounding area (Vannozzi 2007). At its inception in 1818, the San Niccolò constituted 34 patients housed in a building referred to as "Casa del Bigi" (House of the Frustrated), which served as an intermediate reception facility for the patients of Siena and Grosseto provinces, prior to being sent on to asylum facilities in Florence (Starnini 2015). At this time, the institution that would be known as the San Niccolò was owned and managed by the Compagnia dei Disciplinati (Company of the Disciples), who would later become the Società di Esecutori di Pie Disposizioni (Society of Executors of Pious Dispositions), and cared for "occult" pregnant women and children with developmental disabilities, in addition to those with mental illness (Starnini 2015). From 1818 until 1858, the San Niccolò was typical of institutions of the period in which focus was largely on custodial care. The 1858 appointment of Carlo Livi as the first medical director and superintendent of the facility (Starnini 2015) was revolutionary for the asylum and Italian psychiatry in general (Guarnieri 1991), and emblematic of a shift in ideas regarding the nature and treatment of mental illness. This groundswell had begun in the eighteenth century, challenging prior notions of mental illness and modes of effective treatment. There was an increasing optimism that mental illness could be definitively described and understood, and from this knowledge, cured (Eghigian 2010; Shorter 1997). Growing out of this eighteenth-century curative optimism and the rise of the importance of asylums, practitioners—especially of the nineteenth century—started to view the asylum *itself* as curative (Shorter 1997), drawing on the ideas of William Battie, Vincenzo Chiarugi, Philippe Pinel, and Jean-Etienne Esquirol. As articulated by Esquirol, the "therapeutic asylum" encompassed two aspects: orderly routine oriented around community, and a strong doctor-patient relationship (Shorter 1997). Efforts focused on creating an asylum routine, to include labor, that encouraged limit-setting and self-mastery in pursuit of the value of self-discipline; Pinel advocated for structuring the day through work specifically, while Esquirol formalized the notion of a daily regime in general as therapeutic (Shorter 1997). This overall movement toward holism and treatment methods considered to be more humane (Eghigian 2010), but with a focus on labor, routine, and strong doctor-patient relationships, was termed "moral therapy" and hinged on notions originally put forth by Chiarugi—ideas that Livi brought to the San Niccolò.

During his time as director (1858–1873), Livi divided patients by sex and diagnosis, championing a "moral treatment" regime that included agricultural work, gendered craft activities, and recreation. This approach was directly reflective of the "therapeutic asylum" and "moral treatment" championed by Esquirol and others. Additionally, he instituted the keeping of patient medical records, established a scientific library, and campaigned for the specialization of the San Niccolò as a center for research (Starnini 2015). Under this era of "moral treatment" and increasing specialization, patient populations grew from 159 in 1858 to over 800 in 1873, unimpeded by the gradual removal of the "occult" pregnant individuals and those considered to be "sickly" (Starnini 2015). Another revolutionary change began during Livi's tenure—the collection of now more-plentiful deceased asylum patients for dissection, anatomization, and medical study. This practice, taking place between 1862–1931, lead to the creation of the Siena Craniological Collection. While this practice may seem exceptional or remarkable, in fact, many institutional skeletal assemblages are composed of the remains of marginalized individuals used for medical study, dissection, and anatomization, a trend that is directly reflective of institutionalization laws, socioeconomic stratification, and historical beliefs regarding the dead body and proper postmortem treatment.

Institutionalization Laws

Italian psychiatry and psychiatric treatment throughout the later nineteenth and twentieth centuries are characterized by a complex and intertwined relationship with criminology and the legal system (Traverso, Ciappi, and Ferracuti 2000). Indeed, evolving thought regarding the status and treatment of the mentally ill are reflected in changes in the legal code throughout time (Di Lorito et al. 2017; Traverso, Ciappi, and Ferracuti 2000). Italian views and treatment of the mentally ill stress a need to assess the danger a mentally ill individual poses to themselves, but more importantly to society, and to what degree they are responsible for their actions, criminal or otherwise. In such an approach, "danger" might be used to discriminate against the socially deviant (Mellyn 2014).

In the early nineteenth century, regulation of individuals considered to be criminally insane was heavily influenced by Article 64 of the Napoleonic Penal Code, which posits a lack of responsibility due to dementia or compulsion that the individual could not resist (Traverso, Ciappi, and Ferracuti 2000). This premise allowed for the growth of psychiatry in general, and forensic psychiatry in particular, as there was now a need to diagnose the mental illnesses referred to by Article 64. Partially reflecting these early views, during the initial period when the collection of San Niccolò patient remains was taking place, the hospital followed the popular principal of "moral treatment" in which mental illness could be treated primarily using work and distraction (Vannozzi 2007), as discussed previously. Both Article 64 and the early treatment approach at the San Niccolò are reflective of classical social philosophical beliefs that emphasize free will, as opposed to innate mental illness or criminality (Di Lorito et al. 2017). The so-called "Classical School" had influenced criminal policies throughout Europe since 1750 and was associated in Italy with the writings of Cesare Beccaria (Traverso, Ciappi, and Ferracuti 2000). In the second half of the nineteenth century, the classicists were challenged by the emergence of the "Italian School" of anthropological criminology, led by Cesare Lombroso. The rise of the "Italian School" resulted from increased positivist beliefs among psychiatric practitioners and put forth the idea of the "dangerous individual," characterized by innate/inherited mental illness and criminality (Di Lorito et al. 2017; Traverso, Ciappi, and Ferracuti 2000). Relying on ideals of both biological and social Darwinism, Lombroso asserted that criminals were biologically and genetically less evolved, with instinctive impulses to commit crime (Di Lorito et al. 2017). These changes in psychiatric thought reflect the general rise of biological psychiatry, to include the idea of mental illness as heritable. Supporting the positivist or Italian model, Enrico Ferri, a follower of Lombroso, advocated for the creation of state-sponsored asylums to separate those identified as innately criminal from society in order to preserve public safety. In this regard, an important distinction between classical and positivist thought is the right of authorities to imprison those identified as criminals. Under the classical model, individuals can only be imprisoned or punished for actions or crimes already committed; the positivist school seeks to imprison those suspected of innate criminality to prevent a *future* danger to society, which has much farther-reaching implications for the mentally ill who have not committed a crime (Traverso, Ciappi, and Ferracuti 2000).

Although differences in penal codes did exist between preunification Italian states during the strife between classicists and positivists, the Zanardelli Code was implemented in 1889, and was heavily influenced by the "Classical School" of criminology. Given its roots in classical criminology, the Zanardelli Code did not address the creation of separate psychiatric facilities for the criminally insane. Rather, the law stated that patients who were assessed as both insane *and* dangerous were to be committed to state psychiatric facilities, until the president of the civil court ruled to free the individual or commit them permanently. While the Zanardelli Code was a triumph for the classicists, the success was quickly undone in 1904 with the passage of Law 36, Legge sui manicomi e sugli alienati (Law on Psychiatric Hospitals and Alienated People), which was heavily positivist (Traverso,

Ciappi, and Ferracuti 2000). Under Law 36, admission to a state psychiatric facility was determined by a *pretore* (judge) and relied on the provision of a medical certificate and a request that the individual be committed. The premise of voluntary commitment based on a request made by the patient did not yet exist, and would remain an alien concept in Italian psychiatry until 1968 (Traverso, Ciappi, and Ferracuti 2000). Under Law 36, requests could be made by relatives of the patient or *any other person* with concerns for the insane and larger society (Traverso, Ciappi, and Ferracuti 2000). Patients could be temporarily committed solely with a medical certificate verifying a psychiatric diagnosis, giving the magistrate three days to "validate" the individual's confinement. Although the law strictly required the medical certificate to temporarily commit an individual, in practice, this requirement was infrequently followed (Traverso, Ciappi, and Ferracuti 2000). Following a month of involuntary commitment, patients were relieved of their civil capabilities through a court action requested by the psychiatric hospital director (Traverso, Ciappi, and Ferracuti 2000). Following this deprivation of civil power, the patients were permanently confined. In the rare case of those who were dismissed from psychiatric facilities, record of their commitment would appear on their criminal record (Traverso, Ciappi, and Ferracuti 2000). Law 36 and positivist notions of criminality and dangerousness continued with the passage of the Rocco Code in 1930, shortly after which collection of San Niccolò patient remains ceased.

Structural Violence and Living Agency

In order to understand discriminatory systems of power, such as the system in this case, many anthropological scholars have turned to structural violence as a framework (Armelagos, Carlson, and Van Gerven 1982; Baker and Agarwal 2017; Buikstra 1977; Carlson and Van Gerven 1977, 1979; Goodman and Leatherman 1998; Stojanowski and Duncan 2015; Wiley and Cullin 2016; Zuckerman and Armelagos 2011); although the application in bioarchaeology is more recent (Bright 2021; de la Cova 2012; Geber 2015; Klaus 2012; Kohler and Kramer Turner 2006; Martin 1997; Martin, Harrod, and Fields 2010). Structural violence is used to describe cultural, governmental, and social structures that stymie individual agency (Galtung 1969) in particular how political-economic processes lead to largely accepted systems of marginalization with observable negative consequences. These prejudicial structures then prevent individuals, disadvantaged groups, and larger societies from reaching their full potential, socially, economically, or biologically. It is also helpful to return to the definition furnished by Galtung (1993, 106), in which structural violence is seen as "avoidable impairment of fundamental human needs or the impairment of human life which lowers the actual degree to which someone is able to meet their needs below that which would otherwise be possible." Within this definition, it is important to note that structural violence is framed as avoidable and focuses on questions of *fundamental human needs*. Building further upon this definition, structural violence demands that the analyst consider cultural and social structures that stymie human agency. In order to fully understand the structural violence at work via the San Niccolò, we need to address who the patients were and who was most subject to Italian institutionalization laws.

Prior work (Berger 2021) shows that San Niccolò patients were generally adults of both sexes, of lower socioeconomic status (SES). The greatest number of patients were illiterate and had lower-status occupations. Comparison to hospital records (Livi 1868) and census data (Ministero di Agricoltura Industria e Commercio 1875, 1914) from the province of Siena for the period of skeletal collecting shows that the skeletal collection is generally representative of the asylum patient population, which is generally reflective of the population of the province. This finding shows that preferential anatomization of a particular group was not taking place; rather, the disproportionate representation of lower SES patients reflects the societal stratification of the time period. In regard to diagnoses, the San Niccolò patient population was overwhelmingly composed of individuals diagnosed with organic mental disorders: diseases of a biological origin which can cause psychiatric symptoms (such as epilepsy, syphilis, and pellagra), mental retardation, and dementia. These diagnostic trends are key and are noticeably different from modern Italian psychiatric populations containing greater numbers of patients with depression, bipolar disorder, and substance use (Preti et al. 2009). Skeletal trauma rates were low; however, this does not negate the possibility that interpersonal violence or abuse could have occurred. Ultimately, these findings indicate that the San Niccolò patient population was primarily composed of "ordinary" people of lower socioeconomic status, largely suffering from conditions of a nonpsychiatric origin. For the San Niccolò, research to this point does not indicate that institutionalization led directly to poorer health outcomes, rather poorer health is to be expected give these patient demographics. Given that these findings do not lend themselves to more traditional bioarchaeological applications of structural violence such as an institution or system directly impacting health, it is necessary to embrace a broader definition. Key to this application is the importance of agency as a component of structural violence.

In regard to institutionalization and living agency, San Niccolò patients are people who were committed without their consent and thus deprived of their agency. This analysis of agency does not seek to question the ability of the mentally ill to make decisions for themselves but draw attention to the fact that they were not even afforded such an opportunity. Committing someone branded them as "insane" both socially and legally, regardless of the source of psychiatric symptoms. A large proportion of patients merely had medical conditions, like epilepsy, which were largely untreatable at the time, or had developmental disabilities. Regardless of the etiology of psychiatric symptoms or the definition of "insanity" as applied in the historical context, confinement against one's will constitutes a deprivation of agency. The overrepresentation of lower socioeconomic status individuals in the San Niccolò is not by chance. Once you were committed, it would be very difficult to maintain your civil rights and freedom, and to "recover" from a stay in the asylum, both socially and legally. A general lack of higher-status individuals does not suggest that those of higher status did not experience mental illness, rather that if they did, they did not receive care in the asylum, and were thus not subject to the deprivation of agency through the cultural system of the asylum. As demonstrated by asylum patient demographics, those of higher status were clearly more readily able to avoid commitment, typically by continuing family-based care. Prior to the "therapeutic asylum," the mentally ill were often cared for by friends and family (Eghigian 2010; Shorter 1997); *however*, family-based care continued in Tuscany (location of the San Niccolò) for much longer (Mellyn 2014). As for the San Niccolò patients, we are looking at individuals who were subject to deprivation of their agency, in this case personal control over the methods in which their *fundamental human needs* were met, due to their status as "mentally ill" persons per nineteenth- and early-twentieth-century diagnostic systems, and who were more likely to be of lower socioeconomic status. Both facets of this identity—mental health status and lower status—fulfill the tenets of structural violence in that the combination of being non-wealthy (socioeconomic status) and mentally ill (culturally defined group) tends to lead to confinement and loss of agency.

Dissection and Anatomization

Next, we need to identify why San Niccolò patients were targeted for dissection and anatomization. This discriminatory process—directly reflective of the patients' marginalized status—is again best understood via a structural violence framework. Focused on the imprint of lived experiences on the skeleton—how structural violence gets "under the skin"—bioarchaeological applications of structural violence have framed human needs in biological terms (Klaus 2012) and considered systems that led to poor health, following similar usage of structural violence in medical anthropological and public health contexts (Farmer 1996, 2004; Leatherman and Jernigan 2014; Weaver and Mendenhall 2014). In more recent scholarship, (Cooper, Heinzle, and Reitmaier 2019; Crist, Mooney, and Morrell 2017; Dougherty and Sullivan

2017; Halling and Seidemann 2017; Muller, Pearlstein, and de la Cova 2017; Nystrom 2014, 2017a) some bioarchaeologists have expanded its theoretical application in institutional bioarchaeology and pushed scholars to consider further how postmortem treatment, especially skeletal collecting, dissection, and anatomization, can be framed via structural violence. In the case of dissection, anatomization, and the San Niccolò, the structural violence was directly informed by religion.

Italy is a largely Catholic country—as of the year 2000, 85 percent of Italians identify as Catholic (Boyd and McGuire 2003). Given the primacy of the Catholic Church in Italian history (Boyd and McGuire 2003)—politically, economically, and culturally—the importance of Catholicism in Italy in the nineteenth and twentieth centuries cannot be overstated. With this historical background in mind, it is reasonable to assume that the majority of San Niccolò patients were likely Catholic, and therefore shared ideas about the dead body and burial practices with other Catholics. Christian belief, especially among Catholics, stress the sanctity of the body as a creation of God, in which the individual is viewed as a totality; the soul and body are not separate or divisible entities for the purpose of resurrection (Marrow and McElwain 2003). Ultimately, resurrection and salvation hinge on the performance of the proper liturgical rites at the time of death (New Catholic Encyclopedia 2003), and the maintenance of the body as a complete, unviolated entity (Tomasini 2017). The use of dissection historically as a deterrent to crime relied on these beliefs regarding resurrection, in which dissection—including anatomization (transformation of the body into an anatomical specimen)—robs the individual of the chance of salvation (Tomasini 2017). Anatomization should be understood as a "step beyond" mere dissection in which dissection is viewed as a posthumous punishment or transgression in pursuit of medical knowledge; however, dissected individuals or dismembered components might still be buried, albeit in a non-referential manner after medical use (Nystrom 2017a). Individuals who were anatomized and whose remains—in whole or in part—were *curated* for medical education, were further denied the opportunity for burial.

These negative views rooted in Christian belief did not negate the need for bodies; therefore, various rules and regulations were passed, the most prominent examples in the United States and in the UK, that allowed for the collection and use of bodies of executed criminals, the indigent, unclaimed decedents, and the institutionalized, including the mentally ill. In the case of the San Niccolò, the potential pool of bodies was now even greater due to the increase in the patient population under "moral treatment." Due to the extremely stratified nature of society in the eighteenth and nineteenth centuries, marginalized individuals, including the institutionalized, lacked the agency and resources to protest, resist, or curb the usage of their dead bodies for dissection and medical study (Nystrom 2014; Nystrom et al. 2017). Following this usage for medical education purposes, the marginalized dead were often disposed of in non-archaeological mortuary contexts, to include non-referential disposal and/or usage in museum display (Muller and Butler 2018), reflecting the prejudice of medical professionals and other members of higher socioeconomic classes and a lack of respect for the bodies of "lesser classes" (Blakely 1997; Crist, Mooney, and Morrell 2017; Harrington and Blakely 1995; Nystrom 2014). In many of these cases, (Crist, Mooney, and Morrell 2017; de la Cova 2021; Dittmar and Mitchell 2019; Dougherty and Sullivan 2017; Geber 2015, 2016a, 2016b; Geber and Murphy 2012; Halling and Seidemann 2017; Humphrey 1973; Muller, Pearlstein, and de la Cova 2017; Nystrom 2014, 2017a, 2017b; Nystrom et al. 2017; Stevens et al. 2018), it is the postmortem usage of remains of the institutionalized or underprivileged that has led to the preservation of skeletal assemblages, in which the collection of the dead directly reflects the lack of past respect for the living. This work stresses the link between marginalized populations, and the postmortem treatment of their remains, through anatomization and dissection, at the hands of various institutions, in which dissection and anatomization was viewed as negative, and even punitive. Social capital and socioeconomic status played key roles in determining the collectors versus the collected. In these contexts, including the San Niccolò, postmortem treatment of marginalized bodies serves to perpetuate and perpetrate structurally violent processes, including through the deprivation of postmortem agency.

Postmortem Agency and Taphonomy

Third, we need to understand what happened to the remains of San Niccolò patients after they were anatomized. Current information regarding institutionalization and anatomization suggests that San Niccolò patients did not have any method for consenting to autopsy and anatomization, leading to their preservation as disembodied crania. Taphonomic analyses—the study of postmortem skeletal changes—tell us how the remains of these patients were treated directly and long after death, particularly the ways in which this treatment reflects the transformation of skeletal individuals from people to objects not worthy of respect; how structural violence has played out via postmortem treatment. Beyond being anatomized without their consent, original preparation methods have led to intense decomposition staining (including persistent grease, adipocere, and odor), autopsy that was also potentially against patient wishes, and prolific marking with ink and wax crayon. Modern curation of the remains in metal cabinets has led to further damage and degradation including a large degree of shelf wear and breakage of dentition, and the accumulation of prolific amounts of dust, as well as the presence of insect remains, cobwebs, and mold. Overall, there has been a general lack of care and respect for asylum patients' remains postmortem, both in original skeletal preparation and subsequent management, storage, and use. Since bodies are important within a social system (Nystrom 2014; Scheper-Hughes 2011), postmortem treatment should also be considered from a human rights and ethical standpoint, because the remains still constitute a person, not just a "thing."

For the San Niccolò, "proper burial," directly informed by Catholicism, could be framed as a *fundamental human need*, where infringement on this need entails further structural violence. Anatomization and subsequent curation as disembodied crania are violations of the body as a complete, God-created entity. These violations rob individuals seen as "lesser" (lower SES, mentally ill) of the chance of salvation (Tomasini 2017), as well as proper liturgical rites. For Catholics, both the violation of the physical body and the lack of a "proper" burial constitute structural violence, in which actions preventing salvation could be seen as infringing upon a *fundamental*, albeit religiously constructed, need. These actions can be further framed as structural violence in that the infringement upon the above fundamental need is primarily perpetrated against lower SES, mentally ill individuals confined to the asylum. Furthermore, continued ill-treatment and curation as "things," whose humanity has often been forgotten, also transgresses more modern conceptions of the Catholic body, in that "whatever form human remains take, they are due Christian respect as the final form of the flesh and blood person who lived and died and will rise in relationship with God" (New Catholic Encyclopedia 2003, 360). Consideration of this postmortem treatment also encompasses memory and the current role the skeletal assemblage plays.

Memory and Stewardship

Lastly, we should consider how the asylum currently "survives"—both the skeletal collection and the asylum campus itself. Following Livi's departure in 1873, the San Niccolò was directed by two of his students: Ugo Palmerini (1873–1877) and Paolo Funaioli (1877–1907), and underwent the construction of new buildings designed by Francesco Azzurri, which saw the asylum transformed into a mental hospital "village" containing specific departments, accommodations by sex, and facilities such as rooms for the study of anatomy and secluded "villas" for paying patients (Lenza 2017; Starnini 2015). Under Funaioli, a clinic for the study of mental illnesses was established in 1887, which legitimized the San Niccolò as a research institute and allowed formal study to be carried out at the facility, as opposed to previous medical accreditation at asylums in Florence (Starnini 2015). Additionally, Funaioli began to confront the overcrowding of asylums typical of the later nineteenth and early twentieth century and made organizational changes to the San Niccolò facilities in order to cope with the problem (Starnini 2015). Antonio D'Ormea served as asylum director from 1909 to 1952, but was the first to also not occupy the position of superintendent—whose role was to oversee teaching and research at the facility (Starnini 2015). During his tenure, D'Ormea sought to reorganize the San Niccolò through the transfer of the neuropathological clinic to the civic hospital, as well as the creation of a pedagogical institute specifically for child patients and a mental health advisory center open to all citizens (Starnini 2015). Following D'Ormea's directorship in the mid-20th century, the San Niccolò was subject to the changing legislation and bureaucracy governing Italian asylums, culminating in the deinstitutionalization movement of the 1970s (Eghigian 2010; Shorter 1997) and shuttering of the asylum in 1999, following a long period of closure preparations (Di Lorito et al. 2017; Starnini 2015).

Following closure of the asylum, ownership of the asylum campus passed to the University of Siena. Many buildings from the asylum "village" survive; patient remains (largely crania) are housed and maintained by the Università di Siena—Museo Anatomico "Leonetto Comparini," while archival records besides the collection catalogs are held by Le Soprintendenze Archivistiche (Archival Superintendencies) and maintained by the Museo della Società di Esecutori di Pie Disposizioni (Museum of the Society of Executors of Pious Dispositions) in Siena. The majority of these buildings have been converted to house various university departments including physics, engineering, archaeology, and others. In regard to "site preservation," the previous use of the asylum is still very apparent, but also represents a hybrid environment in which layout, signage, and exterior building appearance maintain some connection to the past, while the interior—the "peopling"—of these buildings is markedly changed. Although there are no efforts to conceal the previous history of these buildings, and therefore the presence of the asylum, it is clear that reuse largely takes precedence over preservation or curation for educational or tourism purposes.

For those interested in the history of the asylum campus, a smartphone application developed by individuals from the University of Siena, titled *San Niccolò*, is helpful in some respects. The application provides historic photographs and background information (in Italian) regarding the asylum buildings, as well as a map and an augmented reality feature. Background information also includes audio discussion in Italian, entitled "La voce del manicomio," of each area of interest. In general, this background information reflects antiquated viewpoints of asylum patients, and focuses on historical changes in the asylum as opposed to patients' treatment, humanity, dignity, or individualism. Ultimately, the repurposed asylum buildings and the interpretive material provided by the application utterly divorce the site of past asylum events from the artifacts of this life, such as the remains of San Niccolò patients.

In regard to patient remains, while the facility housing archival records is immediately across from the original asylum gate, patient remains are stored at the Museo Anatomico on the San Miniato campus—a lengthy bus ride away from the original asylum buildings on the main university campus. Remains are stored in metal cabinets, with little indication as to their identity or purpose. Although the remains are ostensibly part of the Museo Anatomico collection, they are not presented or curated as such. The Museo Anatomico space largely focuses on historical medical instrumentation, literature, and preserved specimens—with limited interpretive material. School tours of the museum space do take place, but the craniological collection is not truly integrated into the current Museo Anatomico curation approach. Furthermore, the collection is not used by current students and work concerning the bioarchaeological context of the collection has been scant, barring the research discussed here (Berger 2021). The postmortem treatment of San Niccolò patients—the skeletal assemblage and its continued stewardship by the University of Siena—are largely typical of historical anatomical collections and showcase the problematic nature of these type of collections. Considered within a structural violence framework, collections such as the present case study can also serve as a jumping-off point for articulating best bioarchaeological practice. How do we, as scholars, ethically move forward in these contexts given past infringements of agency within a violent, discriminatory system?

A WAY FORWARD?—BIOARCHAEOLOGICAL PRACTICE AS RESTORATIVE

As highlighted by Squires, Errickson, and Márquez-Grant (2019b), to date, there is a general lack of scholarly engagement with and consideration of ethics within biological anthropology, although recent work (Caffell and Jakob 2019; de Tienda Palop and Currás 2019; Gareth Jones 2019; Knüsel 2019; Moon 2019; Squires, Errickson, and Márquez-Grant 2019a, 2019b) has sought to interrogate the dignity of the dead, human rights after death, ethical dilemmas in human anatomy, and the management of university skeletal collections more closely. While highly fruitful, theoretically engaging, and offering some suggestions for research, teaching, and curation, these discussions do not offer *enough explicit* guidance for those considering or actively conducting work with historical anatomical collections. For bioarchaeological scholars, the access point to history is through these people themselves—and the questions of agency and consent loom large. Such an approach makes it nearly impossible to ignore a shared humanity with past peoples and demands that bioarchaeologists use and share their findings in ways that encourage inquiry into modern institutions and systems of discrimination.

GUIDELINES

Building upon prior efforts (Caffell and Jakob 2019; Gareth Jones 2019; Squires, Errickson, and Márquez-Grant 2019a), as well as cues from other anthropological subfields such as medical and cultural anthropology, a set of guidelines is offered below for working with collections like the current case study—practices which acknowledge past structural violence and attempt to mitigate further harm. Many of these suggestions reflect general "best" practices among bioarchaeologists and forensic anthropologists, but especially bear repeating vis-à-vis the use of remains of those anatomized without their consent, such that continued scholarly use can in some way maintain and restore dignity. Ultimately, we must be prepared to answer, via practice, a series of three ethical challenges.

Respect for Skeletal Individuals

First, at all times, the research should seek to protect the identities of subjects, similar to measures taken to ensure participant anonymity in studies of living or recently deceased populations. Individuals should be referred to by curatorial identifier or basic biological identity (age and sex) only—no names should be used even if they are known (as is the case of the Siena Craniological Collection). Researchers should strive for transparency and public engagement in the presentation of their findings, but photos of anatomized individuals should only be published in academic contexts such as peer-reviewed articles, theses and dissertations, book chapters etc. Use of these photos should be limited and circumspect. Although research may be publicized through social media or popular news outlets, images of skeletal individuals should not be used in these contexts. Such an approach has been taken in the scholarly inquiry of the San Niccolò by the author (Berger 2021). No patient names have been used at any time. When limited photos of collection catalogs with patient names have been shared, names have been blurred. Skeletal photos have been shared in limited scholarly contexts, such as the research mentioned above; however, over time the author has tended to omit photographs of patient skeletal remains. Indeed, no patient photos are included in this chapter.

Respect also entails consideration of how remains are stored and handled. Much of this guidance is drawn directly from the taphonomic changes noted on the San Niccolò skeletal individuals. While not atypical of a historical anatomical collection, these changes are not reflective of a stance rooted in respect and dignity for the dead, with curatorial practices specifically aimed at preventing undue postmortem changes and further structural violence. Best practices for storage and handling should include storing human remains separate from other curated items, such as associated material culture. Storage containers, shelves and work surfaces should be padded to prevent damage to the remains. Mandibles should not be stored in articulation with maxillae, to prevent bumping or damaging the dentition against itself. Loose teeth lost postmortem should be stored such that original provenience is maintained.

Although it is understood that historical curatorial methods may have entailed permanent marking of the remains, current practices should seek to limit damage to the bone while also preventing commingling. Any marking for the purposes of research, such as cranial landmarks, should be done in pencil and erased as soon as possible after analysis. Remains should be stored and maintained in a manner that prevents further degradation or unnecessary taphonomic changes such as mold growth, water damage, insect infestation, sun bleaching etc. Curatorial practices should include cleaning of remains as necessary to prevent accumulation of dust, and removal or mitigation of remaining soft tissue or grease which may encourage further decomposition and/or bacterial/fungal growth. Cleaning of remains should seek to balance continued preservation and overall cleanliness without inducing further taphonomic changes, so the use of boiling water and harsh chemicals should be avoided.

In regard to curation, care should also be taken in the maintenance of documentary records. In particular, collections should be tracked using digital records to prevent data loss, in addition to any historical catalogs or registers that may exist. Access to remains should be limited to curatorial/institutional staff, active researchers, and germane stakeholders. Remains should not be removed from the storage and analysis facilities. Research using destructive analyses should be highly scrutinized, and only approved when the greatest data benefit can be garnered from limited analyses.

In the case of the San Niccolò, the author is not the steward of the skeletal collection and has no direct control over its continued maintenance; however, all research by the author concerning the San Niccolò has incorporated these practices if/when they are within the author's purview. No destructive analyses have been undertaken, and prior research with the San Niccolò collection (Berger 2021) entailed the digitization of the handwritten catalogs, in order to enable future studies using this information. Ultimately, offering unsolicited advice to other institutions regarding their practices can be fraught. Less-than-ideal practices are likely not attributable to malice but may be complicated by issues of space, resources, and practitioner training.

The guidelines above are not militantly prescriptive but should serve as outer limits of respectful treatment for skeletal individuals.

Respect for Living Stakeholders

Research and curatorial practice address the skeletal individuals themselves; however, historical institutional and anatomical collections do not exist in a vacuum. Scholars should consider that published research findings may be read by members of the community from which the anatomized individuals were historically drawn, and by those who were the "anatomizers." Consultation with representative stakeholders, such as researchers hailing from these communities, is recommended, even when not required by law or professional codes of ethics. If at all possible, descendants and other stakeholders should dictate the amount and manner of research that occurs.

The San Niccolò provides an example where ideal practice is just that—an ideal. While skeletal individuals are identified, locating, and liaising with descendants would be extremely challenging and costly, even impossible, and has not been undertaken to this point. Additionally, the craniological collection represents only a portion of each individual's remains. The disposition of postcranial remains is unknown. If they are in an archaeological context (which is likely), recovery of the remains and reunification with the corresponding skull or cranium would again be challenging, even impossible. Descendent and other stakeholder interest in the repatriation of remains is unknown; however, the University of Siena is currently the acknowledged "owner" of the collection. While undoubtedly problematic, the logistical difficulty, prohibitive cost, and potential negative undertone associated with bringing the collection to greater light may also reduce the university's interest in repatriation. As the university is the only "available" stakeholder currently, the author's research with the San Niccolò to this point has been at the authorization of the university; however, their approval of *specific* subject matter has not been sought, as this would represent as infringement of the author's intellectual freedom. Nonetheless, treatment of the various topics by the author has always been with an eye to the potential for various stakeholders as readers.

Research as Restorative: Mitigating Further Structural Violence

Lastly, we must consider how research can be produced and not further infringe upon anatomized individuals' agency. Allowing collections to sit unexamined and largely forgotten ignores the opportunity to restore dignity and respect to these marginalized populations through editing and expanding the historical narrative. With this in mind, use of these types of collections may continue, but should be limited to formal study with these specific aims. These collections should not be used for general skeletal teaching purposes. In the case of the San Niccolò, the skeletal collection and asylum history are not part of the narrative constructed by the Museo Anatomico. The current chapter has gathered meaningful information about the history of the asylum and its patients—expanding our vision of the past beyond the picture currently constructed using material culture and archival material. Incorporating this bioarchaeological data into modern conceptions and presentations of the asylum returns humanity, dignity, and respect to past patients. Furthermore, by including asylum patients in the Museo Anatomico in a more meaningful way, there is an opportunity to discuss past anatomization practices and the experiences, both living and postmortem, of the mentally ill in the past. Future research and applied work in this area should consider the larger role of the asylum and its history in the University of Siena and Siena as a whole, and how a more cohesive, "peopled" narrative of asylum history might be conceived of the currently disparate components of the asylum buildings, the *Museo Anatomico*, archival material, and the skeletal collection.

Research can also be restorative by addressing ethical concerns. Publications of research must acknowledge the method through which remains were acquired and the ethical challenge associated with using these remains. Ethics need not be central to every research project but should be included in the background and/or materials and methods sections of publications. The author's research concerning the San Niccolò (Berger 2021) has always followed this tenet, with the current chapter specifically focused on the challenges of ethical bioarchaeological practice, within a structural violence framework.

CONCLUSION: MOVING FORWARD?

The hand of structural violence—the transgressions of consent and agency and the silencing of narratives in our case study—are not rare or exceptional. While helpful for bioarchaeologists, the guidance offered above is a long second-best for the individuals in institutional and historical anatomical skeletal collections—"those whose bodies fall now to us" (Sappol 2017, xi). But it is up to us now—the scholars have become stewards. Now, where will it go? How can we shed light where previously it was dark, provide voices where previously there was silence?

Besides the ethical implications and guidance presented above, scholars who study human remains, particularly those originally collected under questionable ethical circumstances, should seek to make their work meaningful. Bioarchaeologists must undertake holistic work for the benefit of the living. In order to successfully people the past, scholars investigating historical institutions and anatomization practices must incorporate evidence that addresses SES, education, health, and other facets of lived experience—suites of data that are ideally found in human remains and associated documentary material. In the case of the San Niccolò and other historical asylums, bioarchaeologists have more information than past medical professionals or even current biological anthropologists seeking to understand mental illness. At present, there are no biological tests to diagnosis mental illness (Syme and Hagen 2019), meaning no *biological* data pertaining to mental illness is lost by the reduction of individuals to skeletal material. Although bioarchaeologists cannot observe and interact with the past individual during their life, they enjoy the benefits of time, context, and comparison in ways that other analysts do not. Bioarchaeologists can consider change over time, as well as envision the past from a deep time perspective, such as mental illness as a facet of the human experience, as opposed to pathology identified by the advent of modern "science." Bioarchaeologists are able to appreciate context in a unique way, in which place and time are intertwined and ever-informing one another, with the location of study also taking place within the broader space of community, region, country, and more. Too often, archaeologists are criticized for their explicit focus on the past. The example provided by this chapter should serve as inspiration for others seeking to create novel outcomes from bioarchaeological research. We must endeavor to make our work applied, engaging, and interesting to include reimaging what restorative practices look like. This is the call that modern bioarchaeologists must answer. And there is much work to be done.

REFERENCES CITED

Armelagos, G. J., D. S. Carlson, and D. P. Van Gerven. 1982. "The Theoretical Foundations and Development of Skeletal Biology." In *A History of American Physical Anthropology: 1930–1980*, edited by F. Spencer, 305–28. New York: Academic.

Baker, B. J., and S. C. Agarwal. 2017. "Stronger Together: Advancing a Global Bioarchaeology." *Bioarchaeology International* 1, no. 1–2: 1–18. https://doi.org/10.5744/bi.2017.1005.

Baugher, S. 2009. "Historical Overview of the Archaeology of Institutional Life." In *The Archaeology of Institutional Life*, edited by A. M. Belsaw, J. G. Gibb, O. Lindauer, E. Conlin Casella, D. L. Rotman and L. De Cunzo, 5–13. Tuscaloosa: The University of Alabama Press.

Berger, Jacqueline M. 2021. "Of Body and Mind: Bioarchaeological Analysis of Nineteenth and Early Twentieth Century: Anatomization and Institutionalization in Siena, Italy." University of South Florida.

Blakely, R. L. 1997. "A Clandestine Past: Discovery at the Medical College of Georgia and Theoretical Foundations." In *Bones in the Basement: Postmortem Racism in Nineteenth-Century Medical Training*, edited by R. L. Blakely and J. M. Harrington, 3–27. Washington, DC: Smithsonian Institution.

Blakely, R. L., and J. M. Harrington, eds. 1997a. *Bones in the Basement: Postmortem Racism in Nineteenth-Century Medical Training*. Washington, DC: Smithsonian Institution Press.

———. 1997b. "Grave Consequences: Opportunistic Procurement of Cadavers at the Medical College of Georgia." In *Bones in the Basement: Postmortem Racism in Nineteenth-Century Medical Training*, edited by R. L. Blakely and J. M. Harrington, 162–83. Washington, DC: Smithsonian Institution.

Boutin, A. T. 2011. "Crafting a Bioarchaeology of Personhood: Osteobiographical Narratives of Alalakh." In *Breathing New Life into the Evidence of Death: Contemporary Approaches to Bioarchaeology*, edited by J. E. Buikstra, A. Baadsgaard, and A. T. Boutin, 109–34. Santa Fe, NM: School for Advanced Research Press.

———. 2016. "Exploring the Social Construction of Disability: An Application of the Bioarchaeology of Personhood Model to a Pathological Skeleton from Ancient Bahrain." *International Journal of Paleopathology* 12: 17–28. https://doi.org/10.1016/j.ijpp.2015.10.005. https://www.ncbi.nlm.nih.gov/pubmed/29539517.

Boutin, A. T., and M. P. Callahan. 2019. "Increasing Empathy and Reducing Prejudice: An Argument for Fictive Osteobiogrpahical Narrative." *Bioarchaeology International* 3, no. 1: 78–87.

Boyd, C. E., and M. R. P. McGuire. 2003. Italy, the Catholic Church In. In *New Catholic Encyclopedia*. Detroit: Gale.

Bright, L. N. 2021. "Structural Violence: Epistemological Considerations." In *Theoretical Approaches in Bioarchaeology*, edited by C. M. Cheverko, J. R. Prince-Buitenhuys and M. Hubbe, 131–49. New York: Routledge.

Buikstra, J. E. 1977. "Biocultural Dimensions of Archaeological Study: A Regional Perspective." Proceedings of the Southern Anthropological Society, Athens, GA.

———. 2006. "Preface." In *Bioarchaeology: The Contextual Analysis of Human Remains*, edited by J. E. Buikstra and L. A. Beck, xvii–xx. London: Elsevier.

Caffell, A., and T. Jakob. 2019. "'The Dead Teach the Living': Ethical Considerations Concerning the Management of Collecitons of Human Remains in Universities." In *Ethical Approaches to Human Remains: A Global Challenge in Bioarchaeology and Forensic Anthropology*, edited by K. Squires, D. Errickson and N. Márquez-Grant, 179–210. Cham: Springer International.

Carlson, D. S., and D. P. Van Gerven. 1977. "Masticatory Function and Post-Pleistocene Evolution in Nubia." *American Journal of Physical Anthropology* 46: 495–506.

———. 1979. "Diffusion, Biological Determinism, and Biocultural Adaptation in the Nubian Corridor." *American Anthropologist* 81: 561–80.

Collins, E. 2009. "An Osteological and Mortuary Analyiss of the Insane Asylum of California Cemetery, 1851–854." unpublished masters thesis, Calfornia State University, Chico.

Conlin Casella, E. 2009. "On the Enigma of Incarceration: Philosophical Approaches to Confinement in the Modern Era." In *The Archaeology of Institutional Life*, edited by A. M. Belsaw, J. G. Gibb, O. Lindauer, E. Conlin Casella, D. L. Rotman and L. De Cunzo, 17–32. Tuscaloosa: The University of Alabama Press.

Cooper, C., B. Heinzle, and T. Reitmaier. 2019. "Evidence of Infectious Disease, Trauma, Disability and Deficiency in Skeletons from the 19th/20th Century Correctional Facility and Asylum <<Realta>> in Cazis, Switzerland." *PLoS One* 14 (5): e0216483. https://doi.org/10.1371/journal.pone.0216483. https://www.ncbi.nlm.nih.gov/pubmed/31067285.

Crist, T. A., D. B. Mooney, and K. A. Morrell. 2017. "'The Mangled Remains of What Had Been Humanity': Evidence of Autopsy and Dissection at Philadelphia's Blockley Almshouse, 1835–1895." In *The Bioarchaeology of Dissection and Autopsy in the United States*, edited by K. C. Nystrom, 259–78. Cham: Springer International Publishing.

Curtis-Richardson, M. M. 1997. "Corpses as Commodities: An Ethnography of Covert Medical Practices in Georgia, Circa 1835–1997." In *Bones in the Basement: Postmortem Racism in Nineteenth-Century Medical Training*, edited by R. L. Blakely and J. M. Harrington, 340–70. Washington, DC: Smithsonian Institution.

De Cunzo, L. 2009. "The Future of the Archaeology of Institutions." In *The Archaeology of Institutional Life*, edited by A. M. Belsaw, J. G. Gibb, O. Lindauer, E. Conlin Casella, D. L. Rotman and L. De Cunzo, 206–13. Tuscaloosa: The University of Alabama Press.

de la Cova, C. 2012. "Patterns of Trauma and Violence in 19th-Century-Born African American and Euro-American Females." *International Journal of Paleopathology* 2, no. 2–3: 61–68.

———. 2021. "Making Silenced Voices Speak: Restoring Neglected and Ignored Identities in Anatomical Collections." In *Theoretical Approaches in Bioarchaeology*, edited by C. M. Cheverko, J. R. Prince-Buitenhuys and M. Hubbe, 150–169. New York: Routledge.

de Tienda Palop, L., and B. X. Currás. 2019. "The Dignity of the Dead: Ethical Reflections on the Archaeology of Human Remains." In *Ethical Approaches to Human Remains: A Global Challenge in Bioarchaeology and Forensic Anthropology*, edited by K. Squires, D. Errickson and N. Márquez-Grant, 19–38. Cham: Springer International.

Di Lorito, C., L. Castelletti, I. Lega, B. Gualco, F. Scarpa, and B. Vllm. 2017. "The Closing of Forensic Psychiatric Hospitals in Italy: Determinants, Current Status and Future Perspectives. A Scoping Review." *International Journal of Law and Psychiatry* 55: 54–63. https://doi.org/10.1016/j.ijlp.2017.10.004. https://www.ncbi.nlm.nih.gov/pubmed/29157512.

DiGangi, E. A., and J. E. Sirianni. 2017. "Maxillary Sinus Infection in a 19th-Century Almshouse Skeletal Sample." *International Journal of Osteoarchaeology* 27, no. 2: 155–66. https://doi.org/10.1002/oa.2526.

Dittmar, Jenna, and Piers Mitchell. 2019. "Equality after Death: The Dissection of the Female Body for Anatomical Education in Nineteenth-Century England." *Bioarchaeology International* 2, no. 4: 283–94. https://doi.org/10.5744/bi.2019.1002.

Dougherty, S. P., and N. C. Sullivan. 2017. "Autopsy, Dissection, and Anatomical Exploration: The Postmortem Fate of the Underclass and Institutionalized in Old Milwaukee." In *The Bioarchaeology of Dissection and Autopsy in the United States*, edited by K. C. Nystrom, 205–36. Cham: Springer International Publishing.

Eghigian, G. 2010. *From Madness to Mental Health: Psychiatric Disorder and Its Treatment in Western Civilization*. New Brunswick, NJ: Rutgers University Press.

Farmer, P. 1996. "On Suffering and Structural Violence: A View from Below." *Daedalus* 125, no. 1: 261–83.

———. 2004. "An Anthropology of Structural Violence." *Current Anthropology* 45, no. 3: 305–25.

Fennelly, Katherine. 2014. "Out of Sound, out of Mind: Noise Control in Early Nineteenth-Century Lunatic Asylums in England and Ireland." *World Archaeology* 46, no. 3: 416–30. https://doi.org/10.1080/00438243.2014.909098.

Galtung, J. 1969. "Violence, Peace and Peace Research." *Journal of Peace Research* 6: 167–91.

———. 1993. "Kultuerlle Gewalt." *Der Burger im Staat* 43: 106–12.

Garcia-Putnam, Alexander. 2021. "Dissected, Forgotten, and Fragmented: An Analysis of Anatomized Skeletal Remains from Charity Hospital Cemetery# 2, New Orleans, La (1847–1929)." University of Wyoming.

Garcia-Putnam, Alex, Christine Halling, and Ryan M Seidemann. 2023. "Postmortem Examination as Necroviolence at Charity Hospital Cemetery No. 2 (1847–1929)." *Historical Archaeology*: 1–21.

Gareth Jones, D. 2019. "The Ethical Awakening of Human Anatomy: Reassessing the Past and Envisioning a More Ethical Future." In *Ethical Approaches to Human Remains: A Global Challenge in Bioarchaeology and Forensic Anthropology*, edited by K. Squires, D. Errickson and N. Márquez-Grant, 73–94. Cham: Springer International.

Geber, J. 2015. *Victims of Ireland's Great Famine: The Bioarchaeology of Mass Burials at Kilkenny Union Workhouse*. Gainesville: University Press of Florida.

———. 2016a. "'Children in a Ragged State': Seeking a Biocultural Narrative of a Workhouse Childhood in Ireland During the Great Famine (1845–1852)." *Childhood in the Past* 9, no. 2: 120–38. https://doi.org/10.1080/17585716.2016.1205344.

———. 2016b. "Mortality among Institutionalised Children During the Great Famine in Ireland: Bioarchaeological Contextualisation of Non-Adult Mortality Rates in the Kilkenny Union Workhouse, 1846–1851." *Continuity and Change* 31, no. 1: 101–26. https://doi.org/10.1017/s0268416016000096.

Geber, J., J. Bergman, and E. Iregren. 2019. "Harvested Bodies: Anatomisation of Adolescent Suicides in Nineteenth-Century Scania, Sweden." Society for the Study of Childhood in the Past, Sheffield, UK, October 30–November 1, 2019.

Geber, J., and E. Murphy. 2012. "Scurvy in the Great Irish Famine: Evidence of Vitamin C Deficiency from a Mid-19th Century Skeletal Population." *American Journal of Physical Anthropology* 148, no. 4: 512–24. https://doi.org/10.1002/ajpa.22066. https://www.ncbi.nlm.nih.gov/pubmed/22460661.

Gibb, J. G. 2009. "Introduction." In *The Archaeology of Institutional Life*, edited by A. M. Belsaw, J. G. Gibb, O. Lindauer, E. Conlin Casella, D. L. Rotman and L. De Cunzo, 1–4. Tuscaloosa: The University of Alabama Press.

Goodman, A. H., and T. Leatherman. 1998. "Traversing the Chasm between Biology and Culture: An Introduction." In *Building a New Biocultural Synthesis: Political-Economic Perpsectives on Human Biology*, edited by A.H. Goodman and T. Leatherman, 3–42. Ann Arbor: University of Michigan Press.

Grauer, A. L., and E. M. McNamara. 1995. "A Piece of Chicago's Past: Exploring Childhood Mortality in the Dunning Poorhouse Cemetery." In *Bodies of Evidence*, edited by A. L. Grauer, 91–105. Hoboken, NJ: John Wiley & Sons, Inc.

Guarnieri, Patrizia. 1991. "The History of Psychiatry in Italy." *History of Psychiatry* 2, no. 7: 289–301.

Halling, C. L., and R. M. Seidemann. 2017. "Structural Violence in New Orleans: Skeletal Evidence from Charity Hospital's Cemeteries, 1847–1929." In *The Bioarchaeology of Dissection and Autopsy in the United States*, edited by K. C. Nystrom, 165–85. Cham: Springer International Publishing.

Harrington, J. M., and R. L. Blakely. 1995. "Bones in the Basement: Bioarchaeology of Historic Remains in Nonmortuary Contexts." In *Bodies of Evidence*, edited by A. L. Grauer, 105–21. Hoboken, NJ: John Wiley & Sons, Inc.

Hawkey, D. E. 1998. "Disability, Compassion and the Skeletal Record: Using Musculoskeletal Markers (Msm) to Construct an Osteobiography from Early New Mexico." *International Journal of Osteoarchaeology* 8: 326–40.

Higgins, R. L., M. R. Haines, L. Walsh, and J. E. Sirianni. 2002. "The Poor in the Mid-Nineteenth-Century Northeastern United States." In *The Backbone of History: Health and Nutrition in the Western Hemisphere*. Cambridge, UK: Cambridge University Press.

Higgins, R. L., and J. Sirianni. 1995. "An Assessment of Health and Mortality of Nineteenth Century Rochester, New York Using Historic Records and the Highland Park Skeletal Collection." In *Bodies of Evidence*, edited by A. L. Grauer, 121–136. Hoboken, NJ: John Wiley & Sons, Inc.

Humphrey, D. C. 1973. "Dissection and Discrimination: The Social Origins of Cadavers in America, 1760–1915." *Bulletin of the New York Academy of Medicine* 49: 819–27.

Klaus, H. D. 2012. "The Bioarchaeology of Structural Violence: A Theoretical Model and a Case Study." In *The Bioarchaeology of Violence*, edited by D. L. Martin, R. P. Harrod and V. R. Pérez, 29–62. Gainesville: University Press of Florida.

Knowles, K. C., and J. E. Sirianni. 2014. "Pauper Diet, Pauper Dentition: An Analysis of Oral Health at the Erie County Poorhouse." *American Journal of Physical Anthropology* 153: 160.

Knüsel, C. J. 2019. "Foreward." In *Ethical Approaches to Human Remains: A Global Challenge in Bioarchaeology and Forensic Anthropology*, edited by K. Squires, D. Errickson and N. Márquez-Grant, ix–xii. Cham: Springer International.

Kohler, T. A., and K. Kramer Turner. 2006. "Raiding for Women in the Pre-Hispanic Northern Pueblo Southwest?" *Current Anthropology* 47: 1035–45.

Larsen, C. S., and P. L. Walker. 2010. "Bioarchaeology: Health, Lifestyle, and Society in Recent Human Evolution." In *A Companion to Biological Anthropology*, edited by C. S. Larsen, 379–94. Hoboken, NJ: John Wiley & Sons, Inc.

Leatherman, T., and K. Jernigan. 2014. "The Reproduction of Poverty and Poor Health in the Production of Health Disparities in Southern Peru." *Annals of Anthropological Practice* 38. no. 2: 284–99.

Leavitt-Reynolds, A. A. 2011. "A Biocultural Examination of Trauma from the Colorado State Insane Asylum Skeletal Collection, 1879–1899." Unpublished master's thesis, Department of Anthropology, Colorado State University.

Lenza, C. 2017. "I Manicomi Tra Memoria E Futuro: Esempi Europei." *Festival Architettura* 41: 82–89. https://doi.org/10.12838/issn.20390491/n41.2017/8.

Livi, C. 1868. "Memoire Originali Sulle Statistiche Manicomiali—Lettera Del Professore Carlo Livi Soprintendente De Manicomio Di S. Niccolò Di Siena, Al Prof. Andrea Verga." In *Archivo Italiano Per Le Malatie Nervose E Più Particolarmente Per Le Alienazioni Mentali Diretto*, edited by A. Verga, C. Castiglioni and S. Biffi, 345–62. Milan, IT.

Marrow, S. B., and H. M. McElwain. 2003. Resurrection of the Dead. In *New Catholic Encyclopedia*. Detroit, MI: Gale.

Martin, D. L. 1997. "Violence against Women in the La Plata River Valley (Ad 1000–1300)." In *Troubled Times: Violence and Warfare in the Past*, edited by D. L. Martin and D. W. Frayer, 45–75. Amsterdam: Gordon and Breach.

Martin, D. L., R. P. Harrod, and M. Fields. 2010. "Beaten Down and Worked to the Bone: Bioarchaeological Investigations of Women and Violence in the Ancient Southwest." *Landscapes of Violence* 1. no. 1: Article 3.

McGloin, C. A. 2012. "Crazy Bones: Evidence of Insanity in the Skeletal Collection of the Colorado State Insane Asylum." Unpublished master's thesis, Department of Anthropology, Colorado State University.

Mellyn, Elizabeth W. 2014. "Introduction: The Tales Madness Tells." In *Mad Tuscans and Their Families: A History of Mental Disorder in Early Modern Italy*, 1–23. Philadelphia: University of Pennsylvania Press.

Ministero di Agricoltura Industria e Commercio. 1875. Popolazione Classificata Per-Età, Sesso, Stato Civile Ed Istruzione Elementare: Censimento 31 Dicembre 1871. edited by Ufficio Centrale di Statistica. Rome: Tipografia Cenniniana.

———. 1914. Censimento Della Popolazione Del Regno D'italia Al 10 Giugno 1911: Popolazione Presente Classificata Per Sesso, Età, Stato Civile Ed Istruzione (Tav. Iv). edited by Ufficio del Censimento. Rome: Tipografia Nazionale di G. Bertero E C.

Moon, C. 2019. "What Remains? Human Remains after Death." In *Ethical Approaches to Human Remains: A Global Challenge in Bioarchaeology and Forensic Anthropology*, edited by K. Squires, D. Errickson and N. Márquez-Grant, 39–58. Cham: Springer International.

Muller, J. L. 2017. "Rendered Unfit: 'Defective' Children in the Erie County Poorhouse." In *Bioarchaeology of Impairment and Disability*, edited by J. F. Byrnes and J. L. Muller, 119–38. Cham: Springer International Publishing.

Muller, J. L., and M. S. Butler. 2018. "At the Intersections of Race, Poverty, Gender, and Science: A Museum Mortuary for Twentieth Century Fetuses and Infants." In *Bioarchaeological Analyses and Bodies*, edited by P. K. Stone, 71–88. New York: Springer.

Muller, J. L., K. E. Pearlstein, and C. de la Cova. 2017. "Dissection and Documented Skeletal Collections: Embodiments of Legalized Inequality." In *The Bioarchaeology of Dissection and Autopsy in the United States*, edited by K. C. Nystrom, 185–204. Cham: Springer International Publishing.

Murray, E. A., and A. J. Perzigian. 1995. "A Glimpse of Early Nineteenth Century Cincinnati as Viewed from Potter's Field: An Exercise in Problem Solving." In *Bodies of Evidence*, edited by A. L. Grauer, 173–85. Hoboken, NJ: John Wiley & Sons, Inc.

New Catholic Encyclopedia. 2003. *Cremation*. Second ed. Vol. 4. *New Catholic Encyclopedia*. Detroit: Gage.

Nystrom, K. C. 2014. "The Bioarchaeology of Structural Violence and Dissection in the 19th-Century United States." *American Anthropologist* 116, no. 4: 765–79.

———. 2017b. "Conclusion: The Anthropology of Dissection and Autopsy." In *The Bioarchaeology of Dissection and Autopsy in the United States*, edited by K. C. Nystrom, 335–44. Cham: Springer International Publishing.

Nystrom, K. C., ed. 2017a. *The Bioarchaeology of Dissection and Autopsy in the United States*. Edited by D. L. Martin, *Bioarchaeology and Social Theory*. Cham: Springer International Publishing.

Nystrom, K. C., J. Sirianni, R. Higgins, D. Perrelli, and J. L. Liber Raines. 2017. "Structural Inequality and Postmortem Examination at the Erie County Poorhouse." In *The Bioarchaeology of Dissection and Autopsy in the United States*, edited by K. C. Nystrom, 279–300. Cham: Springer International Publishing.

Phillips, Shawn M. 2001. "Inmate Life in the Oneida County Asylum, 1860–1895: A Biocultural Study of the Skeletal and Documentary Records (New York)." Unpublished doctoral dissertation, State University of New York: Albany.

———. 2016. "'A Long Waiting for Death': Dependency and the Care of the Disabled in a 19th Century Asylum." In *Care in the Past: Archaeological and Interdisciplinary Perspectives*, edited by L. Powell, W. Southwell-Wright and R. L. Gowland, 125–40. Oxford: Oxbow Books.

Piddock, S. 2009. "John Conolly's 'Ideal' Asylum and Provisions for the Insane in Nineteenth-Century South Australia and Tasmania." In *The Archaeology of Institutional Life*, edited by A. M. Belsaw, J. G. Gibb, O. Lindauer, E. Conlin Casella, D. L. Rotman and L. De Cunzo, 187–205. Tuscaloosa: The University of Alabama Press.

Preti, A., P. Rucci, G. Santone, A. Picardi, R. Miglio, R. Bracco, B. Norcio, and G. de Girolamo. 2009. “Patterns of Admission to Acute Psychiatric in-Patient Facilities: A National Survey in Italy.” *Psychological Medicine* 39: 485–96.

Robb, J. 2002. “Time and Biography: Osteobiography of the Italian Neolithic Lifespan.” In *A Thinking through the Body: Archaeologies of Corporeality*, edited by F. Hamilakis, M. Pluciennik, and S. Tarlow, 153–72. London: Academic/Plenum.

Sappol, M. 2017. “Foreward Ii: The Afterlife of Death.” In *The Bioarchaeology of Dissection and Autopsy in the United States*, edited by K. C. Nystrom, vii–xi. Cham: Springer.

Scheper-Hughes, N. 2011. “Dissection: The Body in Tatters—Dismemberment, Dissection, and the Return of the Repressed.” In *A Companion to the Anthropology of the Body and Embodiment*, edited by F.E. Mascia-Lees, In Blackwell Companions to Anthropology Series, 172–206. Malden, MA: Wiley-Blackwell.

Shorter, E. 1997. *A History of Psychiatry: From the Era of the Asylum to the Age of Prozac*. Hoboken, NJ: John Wiley & Sons, Inc.

Sirianni, J. E., and R. L. Higgins. 1995. “A Comparison of Death Records from the Monroe County Almshouse with Skeletal Remains from the Associated Highland Park Cemetery.” In *Grave Reflections: Portraying the Past through Cemetery Samples*, 71–92. Toronto: Canadian Scholar Press, Inc.

Squires, K., D. Errickson, and N. Márquez-Grant. 2019a. “Concluding Remarks.” In *Ethical Approaches to Human Remains: A Global Challenge in Bioarchaeology and Forensic Anthropology*, edited by K. Squires, D. Errickson and N. Márquez-Grant, 627–31. Cham: Springer International.

———. 2019b. “Introduction.” In *Ethical Approaches to Human Remains: A Global Challenge in Bioarchaeology and Forensic Anthropology*, edited by K. Squires, D. Errickson and N. Márquez-Grant, 1–18. Cham: Springer International.

Starnini, M. 2015. “Aspi—Archivio Storica Della Psicologia Italiana: Ospedale Psichiatrico San Niccolò Di Siena.” Universita’ degli Studi di Milano: Bicocca. Accessed 11/13/2019. https://www.aspi.unimib.it/collections/entity/detail/279/.

Stevens, W. D., C. de la Cova, C. Judge, and C. Young. 2018. “Skeletal Remains from the School of Anatomy, Desaussure College, University of South Carolina.” In *Bioarchaeology of the American Southeast: Approaches to Bridging Health and Identity in the Past*, edited by S. C. Hodge and K. A. Shuler, 197–224. Tuscaloosa: The University of Alabama Press.

Stodder, A. L. W., and A. M. Palkovich. 2012. “Osteobiography and Bioarchaeology.” In *The Bioarchaeology of Individuals*, edited by A. L. W. Stodder and A. M. Palkovich, 1–8. Gainesville: University Press of Florida.

Stojanowski, C. M., and W. N. Duncan. 2015. “Engaging Bodies in the Public Imagination: Bioarchaeology as Social Science, Science, and Humanities.” *American Journal of Human Biology* 27 (1): 51–60. https://doi.org/10.1002/ajhb.22522. https://www.ncbi.nlm.nih.gov/pubmed/24677226.

Sutter, R. C. 1995. “Dental Pathologies among Inmates of the Monroe County Poorhouse.” In *Bodies of Evidence*, edited by A.L. Grauer, 185–96. Hoboken, NJ: John Wiley & Sons, Inc.

Syme, K. L., and E. H. Hagen. 2019. "Mental Health Is Biological Health: Why Tackling 'Diseases of the Mind' Is an Imperative for Biological Anthropology in the 21st Century." *Yearbook of Physical Anthropology*: 1–31. https://doi.org/10.1002/ajpa.23965. https://www.ncbi.nlm.nih.gov/pubmed/31762015.

Tomasini, F. 2017. *Remembering and Disremembering the Dead: Posthumous Punishment, Harm, and Redemption over Time*. Edited by O. Davies, E. T. Hurren and S. Tarlow. *Palgrave Historical Studies in the Criminal Corpse and Its Afterlife*. London: Palgrave Macmillan.

Traverso, Giovanni B, Silvio Ciappi, and Stefano Ferracuti. 2000. "The Treatment of the Criminally Insane in Italy: An Overview." *International Journal of Law and Psychiatry* 23, no. 5–6: 493–508.

Vannozzi, F., ed. 2007. *San Niccolò Di Siena: Storia Di Un Villaggio Manicomiale*. Milan: Mazzotta.

Weaver, L. J., and E. Mendenhall. 2014. "Applying Syndemics and Chronicity: Interpretations from Studies of Poverty, Depression, and Diabetes." *Medical Anthropology* 33, no. 2: 92–108. https://www.ncbi.nlm.nih.gov/pubmed/24512380.

Wiley, Andrea S., and Jennifer M. Cullin. 2016. "What Do Anthropologists Mean When They Use the Term Biocultural?" *American Anthropologist* 118, no. 3: 554–69. https://doi.org/10.1111/aman.12608.

Zuckerman, Molly K., and G. J. Armelagos. 2011. "The Origins of Biocultural Dimensions in Bioarchaeology." In *Social Bioarchaeology*, edited by S. C. Agarwal and B. A. Glencross, 15–43. West Sussex, UK: Blackwell Publishing Ltd.

Chapter 2

Battle for Bodily Autonomy for Children and Youth with Special Healthcare Needs

Anne O. Odusanya

Disability is any condition of the body or mind that makes it more difficult for an individual with the condition to do certain activities and interact with the world around them (Centers for Disease Control and Prevention 2020). There are various disabilities that can impact an individual's social relationships, mental health, hearing, learning, communication, memory, thinking, vision and movement (Centers for Disease Control and Prevention 2020). People with disabilities are mistaken to be a monolith when in fact people with disabilities constitute a diverse group of people with a broad range of needs (Centers for Disease Control and Prevention 2020). For instance, two individuals with the same type of disability can be affected by the disability in contrasting ways (Centers for Disease Control and Prevention 2020). Additionally, some disabilities may be visible to others while others are not so easy to see (Centers for Disease Control and Prevention 2020).

BACKGROUND

A person can obtain a disability in various ways. One way is congenitally or present at birth pertaining to issues related to single genes, chromosomes, or a mother's exposure during pregnancy to substances or infections (Centers for Disease Control and Prevention 2020). An example is muscular dystrophy that involves muscles weakening over time (Centers for Disease Control and Prevention 2022; Centers for Disease Control and Prevention 2020). Another way a person can have a disability is through association with developmental conditions that become evident during childhood, such as autism spectrum disorder, and attention-deficit/hyperactivity disorder also known as ADHD (Centers for Disease Control and Prevention 2020). Injury is another method of how one can become susceptible to having a disability (Centers for Disease Control and Prevention 2020). Examples are spinal cord injury and traumatic brain injury (Centers for Disease Control and Prevention 2020). Moreover, an association with a chronic condition (e.g., diabetes) can result in disabilities, such as limb loss, vision loss and nerve damage (Centers for Disease Control and Prevention 2020). Furthermore, a disability can be progressive (e.g., muscular dystrophy), static (e.g., limb loss), or not continuous (e.g., multiple sclerosis) (Centers for Disease Control and Prevention 2020).

In addition to physical disabilities, there are intellectual and developmental disabilities (IDD) (Eunice Kennedy Shriver National Institute of Child Health and Human Development 2021). IDD are typically congenital and impact intellectual, physical or emotional development (Eunice Kennedy Shriver National Institute of Child Health and Human Development 2021). IDD can impact multiple body parts of systems (nervous system, sensory system, metabolism, and degenerative)(Eunice Kennedy Shriver National Institute of Child Health and Human Development 2021). Intellectual disability, which includes differences in the ability to problem solve, reason, learn and perform other skills along with behavior regarding everyday social and life skills, can present itself before a child turns 18 (Eunice Kennedy Shriver National Institute of Child Health and Human Development 2021). Developmental disabilities is more of an umbrella term encompassing lifelong intellectual and physical difficulties (Eunice Kennedy Shriver National Institute of Child Health and Human Development 2021).

People with disabilities report poorer health and less access to adequate healthcare than their counterparts without disabilities (Centers for Disease Control and Prevention 2020). Sixty-one million adults in the United States have some type of disability (Centers for Disease Control and Prevention 2023). Chances are you know someone with a disability, have cared for someone with a disability, or you yourself have had or have a disability. Disability impacts all of us (Centers for Disease Control and Prevention 2023). When it comes to adults with disabilities in the United States, 12.1 percent have serious difficulty walking or climbing the stairs and 12.8 percent have serious difficulty concentrating, remembering, or making decisions (Centers for Disease Control and Prevention 2023). In addition, 7.2 percent experience difficulty doing errands alone and 6.1 percent have deafness or serious difficulty hearing (Centers for Disease Control and Prevention 2023). Lastly, 4.8 percent and 3.6 percent of adults with disabilities in the United States have blindness or serious difficulty seeing, and difficulty dressing or bathing, respectively (Centers for Disease Control and Prevention 2023). With respect to healthcare access for adults with disabilities aged 18–44 years in the United States, 1 in 4 adults do not have a usual healthcare provider, and 1 in 4 adults have an unmet healthcare need because of cost in the past year (Centers for Disease Control and Prevention 2023). Lastly, 1 in 5 adults with disabilities aged 45–64 in the United States did not have a routine check-up in the past year (Centers for Disease Control and Prevention 2023).

Despite these continuous and prominent health inequities and disparities for people with disabilities, the National Institute for Minority Health and Health Disparities recently announced the decision in September 2023 to designate people with disabilities as a population with health disparities (National Institutes of Health 2023). The National Institute for Minority Health and Health Disparities also released a notice of funding opportunity for novel and innovative research approaches and interventions regarding the intersections of disability, race, ethnicity, and socioeconomic status on health outcomes and healthcare access (National Institutes of Health 2023). The National Institute for Minority Health and Health Disparities acknowledges that people with disabilities often experience a wide variety of health conditions that are associated with a shorter life course and poorer health (National Institutes of Health 2023). People with disabilities face inequality, discrimination, and structural exclusion from programs, practices and policies resulting in obstacles to comprehensive and timely healthcare leading to poorer health outcomes (National Institutes of Health 2023). People with disabilities who belong to one or more other minoritized communities have worse health outcomes (National Institutes of Health 2023). These health inequities and disparities for people with disabilities stem from ableism (Christakis and Iezzoni 2023). Additionally, the U.S. Preventive Services Task Force was called on to ensure its recommendations systematically consider the effects of ableism, discrimination, and negative attitudes directed toward people with disabilities (Christakis and Iezzoni 2023).

The United States has a very disgraceful history structurally marginalizing people with disabilities by perpetuating ableism (Campbell 2019). Ableism is defined as: A network of beliefs, processes and practices that produces a particular kind of self and body (the corporeal standard) that is projected as the perfect, species typical and therefore essential and fully human. Disability then is cast as a diminished state of being human (146).

Entertainment

Dating back to the late 1800s to the 1940s, people with disabilities were viewed as objects of entertainment referred to as "freaks" for freak shows that traveled across the United States (Fordham 2007) often accompanied with informative lectures that were embellished to grab the attention of audiences (Pettit 2012). Freak shows took place in various settings, such as circuses, fairs, shops, and music halls (Pettit 2012). They were given degrading names including but not limited to the Bearded Lady, the Lobster Boy, Legless Wonder, and Elephant Man (Fordham 2007) and were depicted in print media (photographs, paintings, advertisements, and souvenir postcards) (Pettit 2012).

Print media served as a significant amount of income for freaks and showmen (Pettit 2012). Some of the freaks were also viewed as medical specimens (Pettit 2012). For example, in the case of the Elephant Man, the man named John Merrick was subjected to frequent exhibitions that required him to be unclothed putting what was known as his deformity on display (Pettit 2012). Merrick's case demonstrates the crossover among medical practices and popular entertainment (Pettit 2012). Masses of people from all walks of life, including lay and medical audiences, attended these freak shows in fascination of bodies that differed from the corporeal standard (Fordham 2007) (Pettit 2012). People with disabilities continued to be treated like second-class citizens viewed as unfit to contribute to society (American Civil Liberties Union 1999).

Immigration

Additionally, Congress passed immigration legislation to target people with disabilities (U.S. Citizenship and Immigration Services 2020). The Immigration Act of 1882 prohibited access to US ports of entry, and charged a head tax on each immigrant deemed to be an idiot, lunatic, convict, or individuals likely to become a public charge (U.S. Citizenship and Immigration Services 2020). Also, during this time, the Chinese Exclusion Act of 1882 was passed enabling the exclusion of Chinese laborers from US citizenship with penalties of imprisonment, and deportation (Library of Congress n.d.). The 1924 Immigration Act took it a step further by prohibiting entry of all classes of Chinese immigrants and lengthening restrictions to immigrants from other Asian countries (Library of Congress n.d.).

The U.S. Public Health Service (PHS) performed medical inspections of immigrants, primarily at Ellis Island in New York Harbor (Bateman-House and Fairchild 2008). Seventy percent of immigrants entered Ellis Island, where the U.S. Immigration Service and PHS officers completed medical inspections (Bateman-House and Fairchild 2008). These medical inspections encompassed physical examinations, snapshot diagnoses searching for visible abnormalities, or observations of immigrants carrying their luggage following docking (Bateman-House and Fairchild 2008). The officers labeled immigrants suspected of having a disease or defect with chalk marks on their clothing (Bateman-House and Fairchild 2008). Immigrants who were thought to have mental defects were asked simple questions followed by being given complex tests concerning cubes, puzzles or interpretation of events shown in photographs (Bateman-House and Fairchild 2008). Victor Safford, who was a medical doctor and officer at Ellis Island, wrote that "it is no more difficult to detect poorly built, defective or broken down human beings than to recognize a cheap or defective automobile" (Safford 1925).

The Immigration Act of 1907 denied entry to the United States for people considered to be undesirable additions to society, and referred to them as imbeciles, feeble-minded, epileptics, tuberculosis aliens, and mentally deficient (Ward 1907). The Immigration Act included a longer list of disabilities and diseases classified as cause for exclusion, such as arthritis, bunions, asthma, deafness, deformities, heart disease, hernia, flat feet, poor eyesight, hysteria, vascular disease of the heart, spinal curvature, poor physical development, and varicose veins (Baynton 2001). The 1917 Act implemented a literacy test that required immigrants 16 years and over to confirm basic reading comprehension in any language (Office of the Historian n.d.). The 1917 Act also increased the head tax paid by new immigrants upon arrival, and excluded entry for anyone born in the "Asiatic Barred Zone" (Office of the Historian n.d.).

Institutionalization

Starting in the first half of the nineteenth century, people with disabilities, particularly those with mental illness or developmental disabilities, were seen as incurable; they were terribly misunderstood and feared by many (Marini 2018). These factors resulted in people with disabilities being institutionalized with little to no psychological treatment under inhumane living conditions highly subjected to abuse and neglect unbeknownst to families (Marini 2018) (Neier 2019). An example of these institutions was the infamous Willowbrook State School in New York, which opened in 1947 (Parchus n.d.). Willowbrook housed close to six thousand patients, exceeding its maximum capacity of four thousand patients (Neier 2019; New York City Mayor's Office for People with Disabilities n.d.). Senator Robert F. Kennedy visited Willowbrook in 1965 (Neier 2019). He had an interest in institutions due to having a sister suspected to have a mental illness or developmental disability (Neier 2019). He denounced the conditions at Willowbrook referring to it bordering on a snake pit (Neier 2019; New York City Mayor's Office for People with Disabilities n.d.). In 1972, television journalist Geraldo Rivera did an exposé on Willowbrook reporting it smelled of filth, disease, and death (Neier 2019; New York City Mayor's Office for People with Disabilities n.d.). Although Senator Kennedy's visit and the expose generated public outcry for many years, Willowbrook did not close until 1987 (New York City Mayor's Office for People with Disabilities n.d.). The public outcry led to the passage of the federal Civil Rights of Institutionalized Persons Act (CRIPA) (New York City Mayor's Office for People with Disabilities n.d.). By way of express authority granted to the Attorney General, the CRIPA gives the Civil Rights Division of the U.S. Department of Justice the power to bring actions against local or state governments for violating the civil rights of people institutionalized in publicly operated facilities (Office of Juvenile Justice and Delinquency Prevention n.d.).

DISABILITY RIGHTS MOVEMENT AND INTERSECTIONALITY

The closing of Willowbrook and similar state hospitals throughout the United States sparked what was known as deinstitutionalization moving from institutions to community settings (Yohanna 2013). However, people with disabilities, particularly those with mental illness can still be found in deplorable environments or in underfunded community services (Yohanna 2013). The decentralized nature of the mental health system has led to many people with mental illness, especially those who are poor, to be inappropriately placed in jails or prisons (Pappas 2020). People with disabilities are extremely overrepresented in jails and prisons (Pappas 2020; Yohanna 2013). Individuals with developmental disabilities may appear to look less sympathetic or unremorseful to law enforcement officers, judges, and juries which can lead to misunderstanding (Pappas 2020). Additionally, they may exhibit unexpected behavior at the location of a crime scene (Pappas 2020). People with disabilities who are incarcerated have an increased likelihood of their needs being neglected and not being provided reasonable accommodations (Pappas 2020). This demonstrates the high unmet need to train law enforcement regarding communicating with and serving people with disabilities (Pappas 2020).

The impact of incarceration and disproportionate disciplinary actions concerning people with disabilities also stem from the educational system (school-to-prison pipeline) (Pappas 2020). The educational system was not developed to support diverse learning styles (Pappas 2020). The impacts are exacerbated due to the effects of systemic racism (Pappas 2020). The 2020 Government Accountability Office report acknowledged that 40 percent of allotted special education service time was either unrecorded or underdelivered (Pappas 2020). In addition, the report confirmed that students with disabilities were disproportionately disciplined (Pappas 2020). The report noted that students with disabilities constituted 11.7 percent of the school population (Pappas 2020). However, they comprised 25 percent of students suspended from school, 27 percent of students arrested at school, and 23 percent of students expelled from school (Pappas 2020). Although Black students with disabilities made up 19 percent of students with disabilities, they comprised of 36 percent of students with disabilities who were suspended from school (Pappas 2020).

Furthermore, the educational system has its own horrid past in the United States pertaining to people with disabilities (Pappas 2020). In 1970, only one in five children with disabilities received an education (U.S. Department of Education 2023). Several children were denied the right to education and learning opportunities (U.S. Department of Education 2023). Numerous states had laws excluding children with disabilities, including those who were deaf, blind, had an intellectual disability or emotional disturbance (U.S. Department of Education 2023).

For instance, Judy Heumann, a renowned disability rights advocates known as the mother of the disability rights movement, could not enroll in school at the age of five, due to her wheelchair being deemed a fire hazard (U.S. Department of Education 2023). She eventually was allowed to enroll in a segregated education program for children with disabilities (U.S. Department of Education 2023). This experience fueled her interest in becoming a teacher (U.S. Department of Education 2023). However, she was denied her license to teach because of not being able to walk due to her condition that led her to use a wheelchair since childhood (U.S. Department of Education 2023). As a result of these experiences and many others, Ms. Heumann became a fierce advocate for change for people with disabilities (Office of Public Affairs 2023).

She played important roles in advocating for accessibility in education, employment, public transportation, communication, the built environment, and other sectors through the passage of the Rehabilitation Act (U.S. Department of Justice Civil Rights Division 2020). The Rehabilitation Act prohibits discrimination directed toward people with disabilities in programs related to federal agencies, employment, contractors, and financial assistance (U.S. Department of Justice Civil Rights Division 2020). She advocated for the passage of the Individuals with Disabilities Education Act (IDEA; formerly called the Education for all Handicapped Children Act of 1975; U.S. Department of Justice Civil Rights Division 2020). IDEA requires public schools to make free appropriate public education available to all eligible children with disabilities in the least restrictive appropriate environment in relation to their individual needs (U.S. Department of Justice Civil Rights Division 2020). IDEA mandates that public school systems develop appropriate Individualized Education Programs (IEP) for each child (U.S. Department of Justice Civil Rights Division 2020). The specific special education and related services should be outlined in the IEP to note the individualized needs of students (U.S. Department of Justice Civil Rights Division 2020). Particular procedures must be followed, such as the IEP being created by a team of subject matter experts (e.g., parents and teachers) in relation to the child, the IEP undergoing annual review, at minimum (U.S. Department of Justice Civil Rights Division 2020).

Furthermore, Ms. Heumann was instrumental when it came to the passage of the Americans with Disabilities Act (ADA) (U.S. Department of Justice Civil Rights Division 2020). The ADA prohibits discrimination regarding disability in state and local government, employment, commercial facilities, transportation, telecommunications, and public accommodations (U.S. Department of Justice Civil Rights Division 2020).

She was also influential in the adoption of the United Nations Convention on the Rights of Persons with Disabilities that aims to promote, protect, and ensure equal and full enjoyment of all fundamental freedoms and human rights by all people with disabilities, and to promote respect for their inherent indignity (Office of Public Affairs 2023; United Nations Office of the High Commissioner for Human Rights 2006). In addition to these milestones, dating back to 1865, the Veterans Health Administration (VHA) was established to serve honorably discharged or injured soldiers (U.S. Department of Veterans Affairs 2023). The VHA now provides treatment services for veterans, including women and homeless veterans, such as suicide prevention, traumatic brain injuries, post-traumatic stress, and more (U.S. Department of Veterans Affairs 2023). The 1944 GI Bill also provided veterans with home loans, and unemployment benefits (U.S. Department of Veterans Affairs 2023).

Although the disability rights movement is seen as its own movement, it was intertwined with other identities, such as gender, race, and sexual orientation, particularly for multimarginalized communities (Fleischer and Zames 2011). People with disabilities became self-advocates because of the lack of understanding and discrimination they experienced from others (Fleischer and Zames 2011). The power of the Civil Rights Movement and women's liberation movement inspired the disability rights movement (Heumann 2017; Wright 2023; Yohanna 2013). The Civil Rights Movement took place in the middle of the twentieth century with the aim of obtaining equal rights for African Americans, and ending racial segregation and exclusion (Library of Congress n.d.). Intersections among the Civil Rights Movement and the disability rights movement included protests, sit-ins in which the Black Panther Party supplied food for disability activists, driving quotes from Dr. Martin Luther King, and the Civil Rights Act providing the blueprint for the ADA (Newnham and LeBrecht 2020). The Women's Liberation Movement was initially established during the suffragist movement of the nineteenth and early twentieth centuries, and came into fruition in the late 1960s (American

Psychological Association 2023). These women leaders and social activists campaigned for feminist goals to achieve gender equality: equal educational and employment opportunities through government and legislation, freedom from male violence toward women and male domination through social action against pornography, and the overthrow of capitalism, homophobia, and racism (American Psychological Association 2023). However, the Women's Liberation Movement restricted its thinking to the needs of women without disabilities despite that both women and people with disabilities are understood to be minoritized communities (Begum 1992). All in all, the Civil Rights Movement, women's liberation movement, and disability rights movement shared common goals for minoritized communities: obtaining reasonable accommodations, equal opportunities and justice (Carmel 2020).

The connection among these movements is an example of intersectionality. Intersectionality describes how the identities of people overlap (Crenshaw 1989). These identities increase access to protective factors or exposure to risk factors in relation to varying degrees of power and privilege (Crenshaw 1989). The -isms impact the quality of life for people with disabilities when trying to access various sectors, such as education, healthcare, and more (Carmel 2020), in addition to experiencing unconscious bias from health professionals which impacts how people with disabilities are treated (Pappas 2020). Studies have shown that people, including health professionals exude moderate to strong negative implicit attitudes directed toward people with both intellectual and physical disabilities (Wilson and Scior 2013). People with disabilities have high rates of co-occurring health conditions and more healthcare needs compared to their peers without disabilities (Prokup et al. 2017). Individuals with developmental disabilities are more likely to receive delayed care and experience difficulties getting sufficient time with physicians, including being satisfied with their provider's explanations (Prokup et al. 2017).

Disparities and inequities are more compounded for people with disabilities with additional minoritized identities concerning race, income, gender, rurality, sexual orientation, and more (Carmel 2020). For instance, with regard to child welfare, parents with disabilities are likely to be reported to child protective services without just cause based on the dominant false narrative that a person with a disability cannot parent safely (Pappas 2020).

Reproductive Health

In relation to intersectionality, women and girls with disabilities experience inequities pertaining to reproductive health (Center for American Progress 2022; United Nations 2019). There are many human rights violations that women and girls with disabilities encounter, such as infringements on the rights to legal capacity, making autonomous decisions, maintaining control of their sexual and reproductive health, and raising children as well as, forced sterilization, eugenics, and more (Center for American Progress 2022; United Nations 2019; Stern 2020). For example, in the 1927 Buck v. Bell decision, the U.S. Supreme Court upheld Virginia's law allowing state institutions to condition release upon sterilization (Powell 2021). Virginia's statute was based on the idea that people with disabilities were viewed as defective persons (Powell 2021). This idea was similar to sterilization laws in more than 30 states (Powell 2021). By 1970, the number of sterilized Americans, the majority of whom had disabilities, exceeded 65,000 (Powell 2021). Close to all states have repealed laws mandating sterilization (Powell 2021). However, most states still allow sterilization with prior judicial authorization (Powell 2021). Studies have shown that sterilization serves as a standard procedure for numerous people with disabilities (Powell 2021). Furthermore, research has proven that congregate care institutions or facilities, healthcare providers, and family members frequently request sterilization rather than the individual themselves (Powell 2021). When it comes to eugenics, there were laws that prevented people with disabilities from getting married restricting them from creating and maintaining families (Powell 2021). Eugenics is intertwined with ableism and sterilization and ignited discriminatory and restrictive US immigration legislation (Powell 2021).

Both disability justice and reproductive health are connected to the right to self-determination, bodily autonomy, and access to healthcare (Center for American Progress 2022; United Nations 2019). Health clinics are likely not to be accessible nor have appropriate equipment or accessible transportation (Center for American Progress 2022). Reproductive injustice is more pronounced for communities of color with disabilities who have endured heavier hardships due to mistrust of systems, promotion of ableism, and racism (Center for American Progress 2022).

Independence

In the 1960s and 1970s, summer camps and rehabilitation centers were developed to provide a nurturing environment for people with disabilities to thrive (Carmel 2020). These summer camps and rehabilitation centers served as an avenue for people with disabilities to develop relationships with their peers with disabilities constituting relationships among leaders of the disability rights movement (Carmel 2020). Among this group was Ed Roberts who used a wheelchair (Carmel 2020; Newnham and LeBrecht 2020). The dormitories at his college were not accessible which resulted in him having to live in the campus hospital (Carmel 2020; Newnham and LeBrecht 2020). Mr. Roberts generated the blueprint for the first Center of Independent Living (CIL;

Carmel 2020; Newnham and LeBrecht 2020). Now, there are over 400 CILs for and run by people with disabilities outside nursing homes and other institutions (Carmel 2020).

The Rehabilitation Act of 1973 authorizes funding to support independent living programs (U.S. Department of Health and Human Services Administration for Community Living 2023). The purpose of these programs is to foster peer support, self-help, self-determination, individual and system advocacy, equal access to optimize leadership, empowerment, and productivity of people with disabilities, in addition to the full inclusion and integration of people with disabilities into mainstream US society (U.S. Department of Health and Human Services Administration for Community Living 2023). CILs, at minimum, are required to provide the following services: independent skills training; peer counseling; facilitate transition from nursing homes and other institutions to community-based settings, and postsecondary life; and information and referral (U.S. Department of Health and Human Services Administration for Community Living 2023). Furthermore, CILs can provide housing, transportation and personal assistance; psychological counseling, mobility training, recreation, vocational rehabilitation technology, physical therapy and more (U.S. Department of Health and Human Services Administration for Community Living 2023). Another legislative accomplishment, particularly for community living, was the 1999 Olmstead U.S. Supreme Court decision that deemed unjustified institutional isolation of people with disabilities unlawful under the ADA (U.S. Department of Health and Human Services Administration for Community Living 2023).

CHILDREN AND YOUTH WITH SPECIAL HEALTHCARE NEEDS

With regard to children with disabilities, children and youth with special healthcare needs (CYSHCN) are defined as children who have or are at increased risk for chronic physical, developmental, behavioral, or emotional conditions (Health Resources and Services Administration Maternal and Child Health Bureau 2023; McPherson et al. 1998). CYSHCN require health and related services of a type or amount beyond that required by children generally (Health Resources and Services Administration Maternal and Child Health Bureau 2023; McPherson et al. 1998). The National Survey of Children's Health (NSCH) that is funded and directed by the Health Resources and Services Administration's Maternal and Child Health Bureau identifies CYSHCN through a validated five-item screener asking parents and direct caregivers if their child has needs due to a health condition that has lasted or is expected to last twelve months or longer (Health Resources and Services Administration Maternal and Child Health Bureau 2022). The five items are: need or use of prescription medication(s); elevated need or use of medical care, mental health, or education services; functional limitations that limit daily activity; need or use of special therapies (e.g., physical, occupation, or speech therapy); and emotional, developmental, or behavioral problems for which treatment or counseling is needed (Health Resources and Services Administration Maternal and Child Health Bureau 2022).

The 2020–2021 NSCH reported that 19.5 percent of children aged 17 or under had a special healthcare need (Child & Adolescent Health Measurement Initiative 2020–2021). Additionally, 18.8 percent had one current or lifelong health condition while 18.7 percent of children had two or more current or lifelong health conditions (Child & Adolescent Health Measurement Initiative 2020–2021). With respect to functional status, 14.3 percent of children had one functional difficulty and 9.3 percent of children had two or more functional difficulties (Child & Adolescent Health Measurement Initiative 2020–2021). Furthermore, 34.3 percent of children had health conditions that moderately affected daily activities some of the time, and 9.7 percent of children had health conditions that affected daily activities consistently or often a great deal (Child & Adolescent Health Measurement Initiative 2020–2021).

Regarding healthcare access, 36.4 percent of CYSHCN did not have adequate and continuous insurance in the past twelve months (Child & Adolescent Health Measurement Initiative 2020–2021). Moreover, 17.7 percent of CYSHCN had $1000–$5000 out-of-pocket costs for medical and healthcare while 4.4 percent of CYSHCN had $5000 or more out-of-pocket costs for medical and health care (Child & Adolescent Health Measurement Initiative 2020–2021). For children with medical complexity, the barriers to healthcare access are evident pertaining to interactions with providers (Ames et al. 2023). Providers lacking knowledge of disability, not providing appropriate accommodations, eliciting implicit bias, assuming children with disabilities have a negative quality of life, and displaying apathy serve as key drivers of discrimination (Ames et al. 2023). These key drivers can result in biased medical decision-making, substandard care and suboptimal outcomes, dehumanizing encounters, resource rationing, and fatal medical decisions (Ames et al. 2023).

Fifty-eight percent of CYSHCN did not receive coordinated, ongoing, comprehensive care within a medical home (Child & Adolescent Health Measurement Initiative 2020–2021). A medical home is defined as an approach to delivering high quality and comprehensive primary care (American Academy of Pediatrics 2022). A medical home should be accessible, family-centered, continuous, comprehensive, coordinated, compassionate, and culturally effective (American Academy of Pediatrics 2022). A medical home is not a physical place and it extends beyond the walls of a clinical setting or practice (American Academy of Pediatrics 2022). Partnerships with clinical specialists, community resources, and families and acknowledging the family as a constant in a child's life comprise a medical home (American Academy of Pediatrics 2022).

There were 21.9 percent of CYSHCN who did not have a person they thought of as a personal doctor or a nurse (Child & Adolescent Health Measurement Initiative 2020–2021). Close to 20 percent of CYSHCN did not have a usual source for sick care (a place they usually go to first when they are sick, or a parent/caregiver needs advice about their health) (Child & Adolescent Health Measurement Initiative 2020–2021). There were 17.3 percent of CYSHCN who did not receive family-centered care (Child & Adolescent Health Measurement Initiative 2020–2021). When it comes to referrals, it was not possible for 1.4 percent of CYSHCN to get a referral, it was somewhat difficult for 20.8 percent to get referrals, and it was very difficult for 6.8 percent of CYSHCN to get referrals (Child & Adolescent Health Measurement Health Initiative 2020–2021). Lastly, 42.2 percent of CYSHCN did not receive needed care coordination (Child & Adolescent Health Measurement Health Initiative 2020–2021).

In June 2022, to advance the system, optimal health and well-being of CYSHCN, the Health Resources and Services Administration's Maternal and Child Health Bureau created actionable strategies and core principles with input from a variety of experts, including family leaders known as the Blueprint for Change: Guiding Principles for a System of Services for CYSHCN and Their Families (McLellan et al. 2022). The ultimate goal of the Blueprint for Change is for CYSHCN to enjoy a full life stemming from childhood through adulthood, and thrive in a system that supports their families, and emotion, health, and social needs, ensuring their autonomy, independence, dignity, and active participation in their communities (McLellan et al. 2022). The underlying assumptions of the Blueprint for Change are: 1) Disability is a natural part of the human experience and does not diminish the rights of people to contribute to or participate society, 2) Racism is a social risk factor that has significant impact on the health of children, adolescents, young adults, and their families, 3) Although CYSHCN require more and different types of services than their non-CYSHCN counterparts, the current system is not ensuring delivery of these services, especially for CYSHCN affected by discrimination and poverty, and 4) CYSHCN are severely more impacted by the adverse effects of inequities and social drivers of health (McLellan et al. 2022). The Blueprint for Change entails four domains: health equity, access to services, financing of services, and family and child well-being and quality of life (McLellan et al. 2022). All of these domains are interconnected with the intent to create advancements in the field at the community, state, and federal levels (McLellan et al. 2022).

The vision for health equity is for all CYSHCN to have a just and fair opportunity to thrive throughout their lives and be as healthy as possible regardless of the circumstances in which they live or were born into, without discrimination (McLellan et al. 2022). Principles supporting this vision for health equity are that: 1) Systemic and structural causal barriers to health equity are removed, including poverty, discrimination, and other social risk factors, and 2) Programs, systems, and sectors that deliver, monitor, and fund supports and services for CYSHCN are created and implemented to improve health outcomes and reduce health disparities for all CYSHCN (McLellan et al. 2022). For access to services, the vision is for CYSHCN and their families to have timely access to easy-to-navigate, integrated, and high-quality health supports and care they require, including but not limited to care coordination, home and community-based supports, physical, oral, and behavioral health providers throughout the life course (McLellan et al. 2022). Access to services encompasses three principles: 1) All supports and services at multiple levels (individual, family, community, and provider) are easy for professionals and families to navigate when, where, and how they need them, 2) The workforce is trained to meet the needs of CYSHCN and their families, is culturally responsive, and reflects the communities and families they serve, and 3) Service sectors enhance the ability of CYSHCN and their families to access services by addressing barriers of administrative and other processes that impede access (McLellan et al. 2022).

The vision concerning financing of services is for healthcare and other related services to be accessible, comprehensive, continuous, and affordable; and prioritize the well-being of CYSHCN and their families (McLellan et al. 2022). Principles associated with financing of services entail: 1) Healthcare and other related services for CYSHCN and their families are paid for and financed in ways that maximize and support a person's choice and values in meeting needs, 2) Investments in social and health service sectors address social drivers of health to increase flourishing and family well-being, and 3) Service and payers sectors adopt value-based payment strategies that advance equity, incorporate continuous quality improvement, and support families by enhancing team-based integrated care (McLellan et al. 2022). Lastly, family and child well-being and quality of life recognizes the need for CYSHCN and their families to be active partners within care sectors (McLellan et al. 2022). The vision of family and child well-being and quality of life is that the service system prioritizes the well-being, quality of life, and supports flourishing for CYSHCN and their families (McLellan et al. 2022). The principles backing this vision are: 1) Families, regardless of their circumstances, can access affordable, high-quality, and community-based services that support the emotional, social, medical, and behavioral well-being of the child or youth and whole family and 2) Health systems place value on the use and measurement of both child and family well-being and quality of life outcomes and health outcomes (McLellan et al. 2022).

Facilitators and Barriers to Physical Activity and Healthy Eating for Adolescents with Down Syndrome

In relation to independence, agency, and autonomy for CYSHCN, a study examining facilitators and barriers to physical activity and healthy eating for adolescents with Down syndrome (DS) in south Georgia was conducted (Odusanya 2018). Children and adolescents with IDD have a higher risk of being overweight than their counterparts (Centers for Disease Control and Prevention 2019). Within children and adolescents with IDD, children and adolescents with DS have an elevated risk of obesity (Ptomey, Oreskovic et al., Weight Management Recommendations for Youth with Down syndrome: Expert Recommendations 2023). Adolescents with DS have an exacerbated risk for obesity resulting from genetic predisposition, which impacts nutritional status and participation in physical activity (Bertapelli et al. 2016).

Additionally, obesity among children and adolescents is more evident in the Deep South (M. R. Kramer et al. 2016; Zgodic, Eberth et al., Estimates of Childhood Overweight and Obesity at the Region, State, and County Levels: A Multilevel Small-Area Estimation Approach 2021). In Georgia, particularly, 21.5 percent of CYSHCN were living with obesity compared to that of 15.3 percent of non-CYSHCN (Child & Adolescent Health Measurement Initiative 2020–2021). Furthermore, the 18.6 percent of CYSHCN reported to be overweight in Georgia exceeded the 15.8 percent of CYSHCN deemed to be overweight in the Southeast (Child & Adolescent Health Measurement Initiative 2020–2021). Although research has shown that adolescents with DS are highly susceptible to obesity, very few research studies have investigated this health issue from an ecological perspective (World Health Organization 2007).

The International Classification of Functioning, Disability and Health–Children and Youth Version (ICF) served as the framework for this study. The World Health Organization developed the ICF to evaluate disability and health-related conditions of CYSHCN (World Health Organization 2007). The ICF comprises categories and identifiers related to Body Structures, Body Functions, Activities and Participation, Environmental Factors, and Personal Factors (World Health Organization 2007). The ICF has been used for various purposes, including but not limited to performing needs assessments, measuring the environment and quality of life outcomes, recording data, and research (World Health Organization 2007).

For the study, thirteen parents of adolescents with Down syndrome and twelve adolescents with Down syndrome (one was nonverbal; aged 10–17) were recruited in two health districts through partnerships with a local Down syndrome society and Special Olympics (Odusanya 2018). In contrast to most studies, and to ensure that both CYSHCN and families were active partners, at least one parent and one adolescent with DS were interviewed for each of the twelve families (Odusanya 2018). Of the thirteen adolescents with DS, one adolescent was nonverbal, so only the parent completed the interview. The average age of the adolescents with DS was 12.92 years (Odusanya 2018). Most of the adolescents with DS in the sample constituting 61.54 percent were in grades 6 and 7 (Odusanya 2018). For race and ethnicity, based on parental responses, 84.61 percent of the adolescents with DS were White or Caucasian. With respect to gender, 69.23 percent of the adolescents with DS were female (Odusanya 2018).

With respect to physical activity, in relation to Body Functions, adolescents with DS confirmed that they did not feel pain when being physically active (Odusanya 2018). There were also some adolescents with DS who stated they did feel pain in Body Structures (feet, stomach, abdominal sides, arms) (Odusanya 2018). Similarly, adolescents with DS reported that they can sustain attention and maintain hand-eye coordination while others claimed they couldn't perform these functions (Odusanya 2018).

For Activities and Participation, adolescents with DS reported that they enjoyed playing sports, such as gymnastics, cheer, tennis, volleyball, dodgeball, soccer, swimming, kickball, basketball and baseball (Odusanya 2018). One adolescent with DS described her enjoyment regarding basketball when asked if she played sports. DS Participant 6 said "Basketball . . . because I get to do drills" (Odusanya 2018). Additionally, managing diet and fitness was touched on by adolescents with DS (Odusanya 2018). Another adolescent with DS discussed how she had to ask her mom for permission to play outside (Odusanya 2018). DS Participant 3 said "Yeah, I have to ask my mom and she says [child's name], let's get your bike [laughter]" (Odusanya 2018). Furthermore, for Environmental Factors, being physically active with family members was classified as a facilitator (Odusanya 2018). For example, one adolescent with DS discussed how she engaged in physical activity with her family (Odusanya 2018). DS Participant 2 said "I go to the gym . . . just me and my family (Odusanya 2018). DS Participant 12 reported that he exercised with his family, saying "Yes, but they kind of get on my nerves" (Odusanya 2018). Adolescents with DS also highlighted being physically active with peers or friends (Odusanya 2018). For instance, an adolescent with DS discussed playing with her friends at their houses (Odusanya 2018). Schools also served as an Environmental Factor as a barrier (not providing recess in middle school) and as a facilitator (providing recess) (Odusanya 2018). DS Participant 10 said "I play basketball, kickball, and with the swings" when asked if she played at school (Odusanya 2018).

For nutrition, specifically for Activities and Participation, in relation to managing diet and fitness, all the adolescents with DS stated that their parents regulated their diet or engagement in physical activity (Odusanya 2018). DS Participant 6 said "Well, I need to ask Mom" when asked if she was able to get food from the fridge when she was hungry (Odusanya 2018). With regard to Environmental Factors, adolescents with DS acknowledged that their parents served them fruits and vegetables at home acting as a facilitator (Odusanya 2018). Additionally, some of the adolescents with DS maintained that their parents did not give them fruits and vegetables at home (Odusanya 2018). When it came to the school setting, the adolescents with DS mentioned that their school provides them fruits and vegetables (Odusanya 2018). When asked if their school provides fruits and vegetables, DS Participant 4 said "We have salad there . . . no we have fruits too . . . yeah in the cafeteria" (Odusanya 2018). One of the adolescents with DS stated what type of food she ate when asked how her family helps her to eat healthy (Odusanya 2018). DS Participant 1 said "They cook food. For example, I usually eat like broccoli or zucchini. Sometimes squash. I always eat some healthy food . . . yes like always" (Odusanya 2018).

Personal Factors (children's preferences) also had an influence on their children's healthy eating and physical activity according to parents (Odusanya 2018). For example, most parents discussed that their children only engaged in physical activity if their child was interested in the activity (Odusanya 2018). For physical activity related to Activities and Participation, many parents reported that their children were involved in sports including Frisbee, capture the flag, kickball, swimming, baseball, tennis, football, dodgeball, soccer, basketball, with most liking dance and cheer (Odusanya 2018). However, parents flagged negative aspects of the competitive sports for their children (Odusanya 2018). Parent Participant 6 said the following: "She played typical tee ball, you know typical um even until she was maybe 8. You know just playing typical tee ball and whatever but then it starts to get faster and whatever and you know she can't keep up. So it's always like she's a little bit too athletic and active for the majority of children with special needs. But she's not fast enough for the typical kids. She's kind of to me in a place in the middle" (Odusanya 2018).

Most of the parents stated that their children's siblings engaged in physical activity with their children (Odusanya 2018). Parent Participant 3 said "Yeah, her brothers especially, they are real physical so they are always trying to get her to go out and play, they are good about it" (Odusanya 2018). However, two parents expressed that their children's siblings did not engage in physical activity with their children because their children's siblings did not want to exercise or were not at home with the children (Odusanya 2018). For Environmental Factors, parents stated that their children's schools provided opportunities for physical activity including recess, physical education, and competitive sports acting as a facilitator (Odusanya 2018). Additionally, some parents affirmed that their children were physically active with their friends (Odusanya 2018). However, there were some parents who stated that their children experienced trouble communicating with peers or maintaining relationships (Odusanya 2018). Parent Participant 9 said:

"But . . . he doesn't have any friends that he plays with around here or that he just like goes to their house and stuff. . . . He doesn't have that kind of relationship with anyone. He . . . kind of separates himself from people he doesn't know" (Odusanya 2018). In relation to Body Functions, parents often mentioned that their children experienced difficulty with hand-eye coordination, sustaining attention, retrieving and processing memory of structured rules when they engaged in physical activity as well (Odusanya 2018). Parent Participant 13 said: She . . . doesn't know how . . . to coordinate . . . kicking the ball . . . they were playing soccer . . . we asked the coach for participation. . . . But the ball comes to her and . . . it's too late or too early . . . not really good coordination. The reaction time is slow, and she gets frustrated . . . wants to quit" (Odusanya 2018). Close to all parents did not report their child feeling pain when their children were physically active (Odusanya 2018).

Regarding nutrition, Person Factors encompassed textural issues and food selectivity concerning adolescents with DS that parents confirmed (Odusanya 2018). Specifically for Activities and Participation, most parents reported that without their management, their children would not eat healthy foods (Odusanya 2018). Parent Participant 3 said "Um, no. She wouldn't pick the right options [laughter]. No [laughter]. Like I said, she would not be able to do anything if it was up to her" when asked if she managed her child's diet (Odusanya 2018). Parents recognized that their children's siblings encouraged healthy eating for their child (Odusanya 2018). For Environmental Factors, with respect to healthy eating, most parents acknowledged food items at their children's schools as healthy food options serving as a facilitator (Odusanya 2018). In contrast, a few parents discussed their dislike of the food options at their children's schools as a barrier for nutrition (Odusanya 2018). When asked to provide their thoughts about their child's food options at school (Odusanya 2018). Parents often stated that they took action to promote healthy eating for their children (Odusanya 2018). When asked if the family helps her child to eat healthy, Parent Participant 10 said: "Yes, just by helping her make good choices and limiting what she eats (Odusanya 2018). You know we don't let her snack all day long and you know you can have a snack between mealtimes, but you can't have 2 snacks between mealtimes" (Odusanya 2018). However, there were some parents who mentioned that they did not promote healthy eating or fruit and vegetable consumption for their children because of time constraints and not modeling healthy eating for their children (Odusanya 2018).

Although parents were able to provide more context regarding facilitators and barriers for their children concerning healthy eating and physical activity, they were not able to provide specific context about the school setting. However, the adolescents with DS reported the items they ate at school along with the absence or presence of opportunities to participate in physical activity. Additionally, parents reported that their children did not feel pain when engaging in physical activity. In contrast, when asked about pain, adolescents with DS identified parts of their body they felt pain when being physically active. This confirms the need to ensure that both CYSHCN and families are active partners in research. Most studies defer to parents and caregivers to speak on behalf of CYSHCN. This infringes on their agency, independence, and right to making autonomous decisions which is perpetuated by ableism. Researchers should intentionally include CYSHCN as active partners in studies as experts of their own lived experience.

REFERENCES CITED

American Academy of Pediatrics. 2022. What is Medical Home? May 23. Accessed August 29, 2023. https://www.aap.org/en/practice-management/medical-home/medical-home-overview/what-is-medical-home/.

American Civil Liberties Union. 1999. American Civil Liberties Union. January 1. Accessed July 13, 2023. https://www.aclu.org/documents/disability-rights-aclu-positionbriefing-paper.

American Psychological Association. 2023. APA Dictionary of Psychology. Accessed August 25, 2023. https://dictionary.apa.org/womens-liberation-movement.

Bateman-House, Alison, and Amy Fairchild. 2008. Medical Examination of Immigrants at Ellis Island. April. Accessed July 2023, 15. https://journalofethics.ama-assn.org/article/medical-examination-immigrants-ellis-island/2008-04.

Baynton, Douglas. 2001. "Disability and the Justification of Inequality in American History." In *The New Disability History: American Perspectives*, 33–57. New York: New York University Press.

Begum, Nasa. 1992. "Disabled Women and the Feminist Agenda." *Feminist Review,* 70–84.

Bertapelli, Fabio, Ken Pitetti, Stamatis Agiovlasitis, and Gil Guerra-Junior. 2016. "Overweight and Obesity in Children and Adolescents with Down Syndrome—Prevalence, Determinants, Consequences, and Interventions: A Literature Review." *Research in Developmental Disabilities,* 181–92.

Campbell, Fiona Kumari. 2019. "Precision ableism: a studies in ableism approach to developing histories of disability and abledment." *The Journal of Theory and Practice,* 138–56.

Carmel, Julia. 2020. "'Nothing About Us Without Us': 16 Moments in the Fight for Disability Rights." *New York Times*, July 22.

Center for American Progress. 2022. Reproductive Justice for Disabled Women: Ending Systemic Discrimination. April 13. Accessed August 1, 2023. https://www.americanprogress.org/article/reproductive-justice-for-disabled-women-ending-systemic-discrimination/.

Centers for Disease Control and Prevention. 2022. Childhood Obesity Facts. May 17. Accessed July 17, 2023. https://www.cdc.gov/obesity/data/childhood.html.

———. 2020. Disability & Health Overview. September 16. Accessed September 25, 2023. https://www.cdc.gov/ncbddd/disabilityandhealth/disability.html.

———. 2020. Disability & Health Related Conditions. September 16. Accessed September 25, 2023. https://www.cdc.gov/ncbddd/disabilityandhealth/relatedconditions.html.

———. 2019. Disability & Obesity. September 6. Accessed July 18, 2023. https://www.cdc.gov/ncbddd/disabilityandhealth/obesity.html.

———. 2023. Disability Impacts All of Us. May 15. Accessed September 25, 2023. https://www.google.com/url?q=https://www.cdc.gov/ncbddd/disabilityandhealth/infographic-disability-impacts-all.html%23text-version&sa=D&source=docs&ust=1696368084485811&usg=AOvVaw25tHQVe-ibZ-qQkoXLLlCL.

———. 2022. Muscular Dystrophy. October 3. Accessed September 25, 2023. https://www.cdc.gov/ncbddd/musculardystrophy/index.html.

Child & Adolescent Health Measurement Health Initiative. 2020–2021. NSCH Interactive Data Query: Did This Child Receive Effective Care Coordination? Accessed August 31, 2023. https://www.childhealthdata.org/browse/survey/results?q=9412&r=1&g=1000.

———. NSCH Interactive Data Query: How Difficult was it for This Child to Get Referrals When Needed During the Past 12 Months? Accessed August 31, 2023. https://www.childhealthdata.org/browse/survey/results?q=9410&r=1&g=1000.

———. NSCH Interactive Data Query: Including CoPays and Amounts from Health Savings Accounts and Flexible Spending Accounts, How Much Money Did You Pay for This Child's Medical, Health, Dental, and Vision Care During the Past 12 Months? Accessed August 29, 2023. https://www.childhealthdata.org/browse/survey/results?q=9371&r=1&g=1000.

———. NSCH Interactive Data Query: Did This Child Receive Coordinated, Ongoing, Comprehensive Care within a Medical Home? Accessed August 29, 2023. https://www.childhealthdata.org/browse/survey/results?q=9400&r=1&g=1000.

———. NSCH Interactive Data Query: Do You Have One or More Persons You Think of as This Child's Personal Doctor or Nurse? Accessed August 30, 2023. https://www.childhealthdata.org/browse/survey/results?q=9401&r=1&g=1000.

———. NSCH Interactive Data Query: Does This Child Have a Place that They Usually Go to First When They Are Sick, Or a Parent/Caregiver Needs Advice about Their Health? Accessed August 30, 2023. https://www.childhealthdata.org/browse/survey/results?q=9402&r=1&g=1000.

———. NSCH Interactive Data Query: Does This Child Have Current or Lifelong Health Conditions from a List of 24 Health Conditions? Accessed August 28, 2023. https://www.childhealthdata.org/browse/survey/results?q=9254&r=1.

———. NSCH Interactive Data Query: Does This Child Have Health Conditions That Consistently and Often Greatly Affect their Daily Activities During the Past 12 Months? Accessed August 28, 2023. https://www.childhealthdata.org/browse/survey/results?q=9329&r=1.

———. NSCH Interactive Data Query: Does This Child Have One or More Functional Difficulties from a List of 12 Difficulties? Accessed August 27, 2023. https://www.childhealthdata.org/browse/survey/results?q=9254&r=1.

———. NSCH Interactive Data Query: Does This Child Have Special Health Care Needs (CSHCN) Based on the CSHCN Screener? Accessed August 27, 2023.

———. NSCH Interactive Data Query: If This Child Received Care During the past 12 Months, Did They Receive Family-Centered Care? Accessed August 31, 2023. https://www.childhealthdata.org/browse/survey/results?q=9403&r=1&g=1000.

———. NSCH Interactive Data Query: Is This Child Adequately and Continuously Insured; That Is, Is Their Current insurance Adequate and Were They insured for the Past 12 Months? Accessed August 28, 2023. https://www.childhealthdata.org/browse/survey/results?q=9369&r=1&g=1000.

———. NSCH Interactive Data Query: Percent of Adolescents, Ages 10 Through 17, Who Are Obese (BMI at or Above the 95th Percentile). Accessed August 31, 2023. https://www.childhealthdata.org/browse/survey/results?q=9617&r=12&r2=56&g=1000&a=18657.

———. NSCH Interactive Data Query: Percent of Adolescents, Ages 10 Through 17, Who Are Overweight (BMI 85th to 94th Percentile). Accessed August 31, 2023. NSCH Interactive Data Query: Percent of Adolescents, Ages 10 Through 17, Who Are.

Christakis, Dimitri A., and Lisa I Iezzoni. 2023. "Calling on the USPSTF to Address Ableism and Structural Ableism." *Journal of the American Medical Association*, E1–E2.

Crenshaw, Kimberlé. 1989. " Demarginalizing the Intersection of Race and Sex: A Black Feminist Critique of Antidiscrimination Doctrine, Feminist Theory and Antiracist Politics." *University of Chicago Legal Forum,* 139–67.

Data Resource Center for Child & Adolescent Health. 2020–2021. National Outcome Measure 20: Percent of adolescents, ages 10 through 17, who are obese (BMI at or above the 95th percentile). Accessed July 22, 2023. https://www.childhealthdata.org/browse/survey/results?q=9617&r=12&r2=56&g=1000&a=18657.

———. 2020–2021. National Outcome Measure 20: Percent of adolescents, ages 10 through 17, who are obese (BMI at or above the 95th percentile): Georgia vs HRSA Region. Accessed July 15, 2023. https://www.childhealthdata.org/browse/survey/results?q=9617&r=12&r2=56&g=1000&a=18656.

[AQ2]2011. "Deinstitutionalization and Independent Living." In *The Disability Rights Movement: From Charity to Confrontation*, by Doris Zames Fleischer and Frieda Zames, 33–48. Philadelphia: Temple University Press.

Fordham, Brigham A. 2007. "Dangerous Bodies: Freak Shows, Expression, and Exploitation." *UCLA Entertainment Law Review,* 208–45.

Fox, Bianca, Gwendolyn M Moffett, Clara Kinnison, Grace Brooks, and Laura E Case. 2019. "Physical Activity Levels of Children With Down Syndrome." *Pediatric Physical Therapy,* 33–41.

Health Resources and Services Administration Maternal and Child Health Bureau. 2023. Children and Youth with Special Health Care Needs (CYSHCN). July. Accessed August 26, 2023. https://mchb.hrsa.gov/programs-impact/focus-areas/children-youth-special-health-care-needs-cyshcn.

———. 2022. Children and Youth with Special Health Care Needs: NSCH Data Brief. June. Accessed August 26, 2023. https://mchb.hrsa.gov/sites/default/files/mchb/programs-impact/nsch-data-brief-children-youth-special-health-care-needs.pdf.

Heumann, Judith. 2017. Our Fight for Disability Rights and Why We're Not Done Yet. January 10. Accessed September 25, 2023. https://www.youtube.com/watch?v=ABFpTRIJUuc.

Kramer, Michael R., Ilana G. Raskind, Miriam E. Van Dyke, Stephen A. Matthews, and Jessica Cook-Smith. 2016. "Geography of Adolescent Obesity in the U.S., 2007–2011." *American Journal of Preventive Medicine* 898–909.

Library of Congress. n.d. Immigration and Relocation in U.S. History: Exclusion. Accessed July 13, 2023. https://www.loc.gov/classroom-materials/immigration/chinese/exclusion/.

———. n.d. U.S. History Primary Source Timeline. Accessed August 24, 2023. https://www.loc.gov/classroom-materials/united-states-history-primary-source-timeline/post-war-united-states-1945-1968/civil-rights-movement/.

Marini, Irmo. 2018. "The History of Treatment Toward People With Disabilities." In *Psychosocial Aspects of Disability: Insider Perspectives and Strategies for Counselors*, by Irmo Marini, Noreen M. Graf and MIchael Millington, 3–32. New York: Springer Publishing Company.

McLellan, Sarah E., Marie Y. Mann, Joan A. Scott, and Treeby W. Brown. 2022. "A Blueprint for Change: Guiding Principles for a System of Services for Children and Youth With Special Health Care Needs and Their Families." *Pediatrics,* S723–S728.

McPherson, Merle, Polly Arango, Harriette Fox, Cassie Lauver, Margaret McManus, Paul W. Newacheck, James M. Perrin, Jack P. Shonkoff, and Bonnie Strickland. 1998. "A New Definition of Children With Special Health Care Needs." *Pediatrics,* 137–39.

Murphy, Nancy A., and Paul S. Carbone. 2008. "Promoting the Participation of Children With Disabilities in Sports, Recreation, and Physical Activities." *Pediatrics*, 1057–61.

National Institutes of Health. 2023. Announcement of Decision to Designate People with Disabilities as a Population with Health Disparities. September 28. Accessed September 28, 2023. https://nimhd.nih.gov/about/directors-corner/messages/health-disparities-population-designation.html.

Neier, Aryeh. 2019. Cleaning Up The Snake Pit. November 8. Accessed July 14, 2023. https://www.aclu.org/issues/disability-rights/cleaning-snake-pit.

New York City Mayor's Office for People with Disabilities. n.d. Our History: Photograph from the Willowbrook State School on Staten Island, circa 1970. Accessed July 16, 2023. https://www.nyc.gov/site/mopd/events/our-history.page?slide=10.

2020. *Crip Camp*. Directed by Nicole Newnham and James LeBrecht.

Odusanya, Anne O. 2018. Utilizing THE ICF-CY as a Conceptual Framework to Examine Physical Activity and Dietary Behaviors among Adolescents with Down Syndrome. Dissertation, Statesboro: Georgia Southern University.

Office of Juvenile Justice and Delinquency Prevention. n.d. Civil Rights of Institutionalized Persobs Act in Juvenile Correctional Facilities. Accessed September 25, 2023. https://ojjdp.ojp.gov/sites/g/files/xyckuh176/files/pubs/walls/sect-01.html#:~:text=Congress%20enacted%20CRIPA%20in%201980,cases%20to%20protect%20institutionalized%20persons.&text=CRIPA%20does%20not%20authorize%20DOJ,action%20to%20remedy%20systemic%20prob.

Office of Public Affairs. 2023. Justice Department Remembers Judy Heumann. March 7. Accessed July 18, 2023. https://www.justice.gov/opa/blog/justice-department-remembers-judy-heumann.

Office of the Historian. n.d. The Immigration Act of 1924 (The Johnson-Reed Act). Accessed July 11, 2023. https://history.state.gov/milestones/1921-1936/immigration-act#:~:text=The%201917%20Act%20implemented%20a,decisions%20over%20whom%20to%20exclude.

Pappas, Stephanie. 2020. Despite the ADA, equity is still out of reach. November 1. Accessed July 16, 2023. https://www.apa.org/monitor/2020/11/feature-ada.

Parchus, Marilyn. n.d. Willowbrook. Accessed July 15, 2023. https://www.cdrnys.org/blog/advocacy/willowbrook/.

Powell, Robyn M. 2021. "Confronting Eugenics Means Finally Confronting Its Ableist Roots." William & Mary Journal of Race, Gender, and Social Justice 607–33.

Ptomey, Lauren T., Nicolas M. Oreskovic, James A. Hendrix, Dominica Nichols, and Stamatis Agliovlasitis. 2023. "Weight Management Recommendations for Youth with Down syndrome: Expert Recommendations." *Frontiers in Pediatrics,* 1–15.

Safford, Victor. 1925. *Immigration Problems: Personal Experiences of an Official*. New York: Dodd, Mead.

Stern, Alexandra. 2020. Forced sterilization policies in the US targeted minorities and those with disabilities—and lasted into the 21st century. September 23. Accessed July 17 2023, 2023. https://ihpi.umich.edu/news/forced-sterilization-policies-us-targeted-minorities-and-those-disabilities-and-lasted-21st.

U.S. Department of Education. 2023. Justice Department Remembers Judy Heumann. March 7. Accessed September 25, 2023. https://www.justice.gov/opa/blog/justice-department-remembers-judy-heumann.

U.S. Department of Health and Human Services Administration for Community Living. 2023. Centers for Independent Living. September 25. Accessed September 26, 2023. https://acl.gov/programs/aging-and-disability-networks/centers-independent-living.

U.S. Department of Justice Civil Rights Division. 2020. Guide to Disablity Rights Laws. Februry 28. Accessed September 25, 2023. https://www.ada.gov/resources/disability-rights-guide/.

U.S. Department of Veterans Affairs. 2023. History Overview. August 17. Accessed September 25, 2023. https://department.va.gov/history/history-overview/#:~:text=The%20second%20consolidation%20of%20federal,activities%20affecting%20war%20veterans.

United Nations. 2019. Expert group meeting on the intersections between women's rights and the rights of person with disabilities. March 19. Accessed August 4, 2023. https://www.ohchr.org/en/special-procedures/sr-disability/expert-group-meeting-intersections-between-womens-rights-and-rights-person-disabilities.

United Nations Office of the HIgh Commissioner for Human Rights. 2006. Convention on the Rights of Persons with Disabilities. December 12. Accessed September 25, 2023. https://www.ohchr.org/en/instruments-mechanisms/instruments/convention-rights-persons-disabilities.

US Citizenship and Immigration Services. 2020. Early American Immigration Policies. July 30. Accessed July 12, 2023. https://www.uscis.gov/about-us/our-history/overview-of-ins-history/early-american-immigration-policies#:~:text=The%20general%20Immigration%20Act%20of,for%20new%20federal%20enforcement%20authorities.

US Department of Education. 2023. A History of the Individuals With Disabilities Education Act. January 11. Accessed August 2, 2023. https://sites.ed.gov/idea/IDEA-History#:~:text=Before%20EHA%2C%20many%20children%20were,or%20had%20an%20intellectual%20disability.

Ward, Robert. 1907. "The New Immigration Act." *The North American Review*, 587–93.

World Health Organization. 2007. "International Classification of Functioning, Disability and Health: Children & Youth Version." Accessed August 5, 2023. https://apps.who.int/iris/bitstream/handle/10665/43737/9789241547321_eng.pdf?sequence=1&isAllowed=y.

———. 2007. International Classification of Functioning, Disability and Health-Children & Youth Version. Accessed August 31, 2023. https://iris.who.int/bitstream/handle/10665/43737/9789241547321_eng.pdf?isAllowed=y&sequence=1.

Wright, Marisa. 2023. A Shared Struggle for Equality: Disability Rights and Racial Justice. July 31. Accessed August 5, 2023. https://www.naacpldf.org/disability-rights-and-racial-justice/.

Yohanna, Daniel. 2013. Deinstutionalization of People with Mental Illness: Causes and Consequences. October. Accessed July 17, 2023. https://journalofethics.ama-assn.org/article/deinstitutionalization-people-mental-illness-causes-and-consequences/2013-10.

Zgodic, Anja, Jan M. Eberth, Charity B. Breneman, Marilyn E. Wende, Andrew T. Kaczynski, Angela D. Liese, and Alexander C. McLain. 2021. "Estimates of

Childhood Overweight and Obesity at the Region, State, and County Levels: A Multilevel Small-Area Estimation Approach." *American Journal of Epidemiology,* 2618–29.

Chapter 3

They Think I'm Fat and Lazy

The Large Body as Social Failure in Japan

Cindi SturtzSreetharan

The past decade has witnessed heightened global anxieties around the increasing "obesity epidemic." These worries are expressed both institutionally and interpersonally, from the enthusiastic implementation of national "sugar tax" policies to a mother's emphatic warnings of her son's impending illness if he doesn't lose weight. These varied efforts to control weight appear to impact people emotionally, potentially creating feelings of shame and self-blame. This is proposed as a crucial reason that attempts to control weight are not just associated with chronic disease, but also eating disorders, depression, interpersonal conflict, and social exclusion (Brewis 2014; Puhl et al. 2013; Puhl et al. 2006). Below, I investigate how different levels of communication around weight are experienced by people in Japan. Specifically, I am concerned with the explicit national policy that mandates a special annual health exam for people ages 40 to 74 years old; it is designed to detect, diagnose, and ultimately provide guided health interventions for "metabolic syndrome" and cardiovascular disease risk. Japan's explicit health policies aimed at monitoring and reducing lifestyle diseases such as hypertension, dyslipidemia, diabetes, and so on are squarely focused on weight prevention and intervention. This work builds on previous work (SturtzSreetharan et al. 2021a, 2021b) that uses ethnographic and narrative analysis to ask: What is the everyday lived experience of "being fat" in Japan?

In this current investigation, I am interested in whether people in Japan, amid a context of low rates of obesity, feel stress, stigma, and experience being shamed by others due to their weight. In particular, does the mandated

Japanese annual health exam (*metaborikku shōkōkun kenkō shinsa*) contribute to an individual's worsening fat stigma and felt shame because it is an explicit event focused on the biometrics of the body? Drawing on surveys and interviews conducted in Japan, this chapter investigates how weight is experienced by men (n=118) and women (n=16) in Japan. The survey investigated the ways that people change their everyday habits leading up to the annual mandatory physical health exam conducted. In addition, a qualitative thematic analysis of responses to the question "How do you feel judged for your body size?" demonstrates three key findings for the ways men and women experience body size and shape judgment: stereotypical tropes linking large bodies to social failure, explicit and implicit judgment in public spaces, and internalized stigma.

While this chapter reports on the experiences of both Japanese women and men, it emphasizes the experiences of Japanese *men* for two reasons. First, theoretically men are *presumed* to be less affected by social stigma and fat shaming than women but there is little empirical evidence this is really the case; accordingly, men are extremely underrepresented in qualitative studies of fatness and fat stigma. Second, in Japan the rates of overweight and obesity (combined) are higher for men than for women; globally this is an unusual pattern in itself (Brewis 2011). The social implications of that patterning for men will greatly expand our understanding of how obesity is a socially constructed phenomenon and how it is negotiated with ideals of masculinity in particular.

BACKGROUND ON STUDIES OF FAT

Anthropology has long held an interest in the symbolic meanings of "fat" bodies. Much of the work done in the 1990s demonstrates clearly that large bodies communicated positive moral values (e.g., Popenoe in Niger; Sobo in Jamaica; and Becker in Fiji) (Popenoe et al. 2003; Sobo 1994). Through this body of scholarship, we can understand that fatness was associated with positive characteristics, including wealth, health, hard work, marriageability, social support, sexiness, and reproduction. However, more recent ethnographic work on bodies in diverse places, including Guatemala, Cuba, the United States, and Mexico suggests that positive valuation of the large body is shifting and changing (Brewis et al. 2018; Carney 2015; Garth 2013; SturtzSreetharan et al. 2021). These studies grapple with the tensions expressed by people with regard to their lived experiences and the biomedical models of weight, including the ways in which cultural meanings of "fat" and medical concerns around weight are not well aligned. People routinely experience public health and social media messaging simultaneously; while the former focuses narrowly on reducing weight the later focuses on thinness.

Taken together, research shows that these social discourses reinforce increasingly internalized messages that weight is dangerous and must be avoided or controlled (Austin 1999; Hardin et al. 2018; LeBesco 2011; Monaghan et al. 2013; Scagliusi et al. 2020; Sanabria and Yates-Doerr 2015; Ulian et al. 2023). Consequently, a context wherein vigilance of one's own body and weight becomes normalized ultimately becomes internalized as anti-fat sentiment or fat stigma. Globally people have come to internalize and normalize body ideals that favor a slim figure that is fit (Brewis et al. 2018); the normalization means that people are willing to go to great lengths to keep their body ordered, which typically means slim and fit. And, people take personal or individual responsibility for their bodies, blaming themselves for gaining weight or valorizing themselves for losing weight. This individual sense of responsibility takes on overtones of personal qualities linked tightly to ideas about self-management, discipline, and morality (Lupton 2013). This highly vigilant, self-aware person is often called a "biocitizen" doing their best for their national body (Costa 2021; Rose and Novas 2007), keeping fit and in step with body norms and ideals just like all of their peers should be doing. The mandatory annual metabolic syndrome checkup is also an example of biopower (Foucault 1990) as the Japanese national government has charged employers with executing the special physical exam and reporting results to the national occupational health and safety agency. In other words, there is national surveillance of the individual body (biopower) in addition to the individual vigilance (biocitizen) people exert on their own and others' bodies with regard to weight and size.

While there is an increasing body of scholarship which looks at the experience of anti-fat sentiment and stigma in the global north (Anderson-Fye and Brewis 2017; Brewis and Wutich 2015; Brewis et al. 2016; Trainer et al. 2016), the lived experience of anti-fat sentiment and stigma in Japan is just emerging (SturtzSreetharan and Brewis 2019; Trainer et al. 2022; SturtzSreetharan et al. 2021). In addition, the bulk of the scholarship on fat and fat stigma focuses on women's experiences (Brewis 2014). Studies that investigate the lived experiences of men with regard to fat and fat stigma are increasing (Monaghan 2005, 2007, 2008). However, recent scholarship demonstrates that men in the United States, too, experience fat shaming and stigma and suffer negative health outcomes including depression and social isolation (Puhl and Heuer 2009; Trainer et al. 2021; SturtzSreetharan et al. 2018; Westermann et al. 2015; Himmelstein et al. 2018). Our own research with Japanese women reveals that they experience fat stigma as a result of interactions with social media, family members, and peers. But, the relationship of public health policies to stigma in the Japanese context requires further investigation.

Worry and concern about weight is rooted in the ways classification of bodies shift and change as people move between contexts (work, school, family, physician offices) and between social networks (coworkers, peers, schoolmates, kin). Norms and evaluations of bodies are socially constructed and discursively maintained. Moreover, people in both the United States and Japan are inundated with surprisingly similar streams of information on the importance and apparent simplicity of weight reduction, healthful eating, and physical activity. However, the broader science of obesity makes clear that weight increases among humans worldwide are due to large ecological, technological, and economic transitions that have profoundly changed our everyday lives, including where and how we work and where and how we procure food (Popkin and Gordon-Larsen 2004; Popkin et al. 2012). Consequently, the ways in which people talk about weight typically include narratives of personal failure such as a lack of discipline, poor nutrition, or lack of exercise; research in the United States attests to this and our work in Japan suggests the possibility of similar narratives (Puhl et al. 2015; SturtzSreetharan et al. 2019).

WHY JAPAN?

Japan boasts one of the lowest adult obesity rates in the modern world, at just 4.3 percent, with a 27.2 percent rate of overweight. In part, these low rates reflect the ongoing influence of the traditional Japanese diet in everyday life, a diet characterized by fresh vegetables and high-quality proteins like fish. While Japan has been identified as a country of extreme thin-idealism, in what may appear contradictory to this characterization, the government of Japan recently announced that the nation is in the midst of a burgeoning obesity crisis. As noted above, the government has taken dramatic steps to do something about this crisis. The "*metabo* law" passed in 2008 specified allowable waist and hip circumferences as well as allowable maximums for other metabolic disease indicators including blood pressure among other screenings. Individuals who are identified as being at risk for metabolic disease face the prospect of health education and counseling classes, periodic health exam check-ins, and weight-loss support services (Manzenreiter 2012; Borovoy 2015).

HEALTH POLICIES TARGETING OBESITY

Japan has a long history of public health policies which serve to shape both institutions as well as cultural beliefs and values (Garon 1997). Healthcare is found across many sectors of Japanese life, most profoundly perhaps in compulsory education curriculum (Lewis 1995; Borovoy 2017). As such, the idea that the government has a role in protecting people's health, broadly defined, is expected (Borovoy 2017). Japan achieves its highly successful public health mandates through a combination of approaches including food education (*shokuiku*), standardized recommendations for health and body metrics, and high values placed on cultural homogeneity (Borovoy and Roberto 2012). Borovoy's work on public health, specifically metabolic syndrome and food education, is located in Tokyo companies, with interviews being done with public health nurses, human resource managers, physicians, and representatives of the companies' health insurance organization (Borovoy et al. 2015; Borovoy 2015, 2017). Scholarship on public health and health policies in Japan, specifically metabolic syndrome and food education, has been focused on the institutional side—companies, human resource managers, physicians, nurses, and insurance employees (Borovoy et al. 2015; Borovoy 2015, 2017; Borovoy and Li Zhang 2017).Work on health policies and dietary problems in Japan have shown that there is a high value placed on eating breakfast as well as the sharing of meals and the important role of fathers in these meal times. But, fathers are often absent from home meals due to busy schedules, opting instead for cheap high-caloric fast food near their place of work, eating with workmates, or eating alone (Melby 2014; SturtzSreetharan et al. 2019). This current study proposes to examine the other side of the public health equation with regard specifically to obesity/metabolic syndrome by talking to everyday men about their experiences with being overweight, health policy, and stigma in Japan.

The classification of weight used in medical contexts relies on the body mass index (BMI). It should be noted that there are many critiques of BMI as a measure of body mass (Adams 2016; Jutel 2006). In Japan, in 2006, the government lowered the obesity threshold from a BMI ≥30 to a BMI ≥25, given the potential health risks for East Asian populations at lower BMIs (Manzenreiter 2012). By doing so, the obesity rate in Japan rose dramatically from 4.3 percent (BMI≥30) to 26.4 percent (BMI≥25). Subsequently, in 2008, the Japanese Ministry of Health, Labor, and Welfare implemented the annual metabolic health check-up for all citizens between the ages of 40 and 74, focusing on body metabolism, weight conditions, and lifestyle habits specifically (Manzenreiter 2012). This *metabo* health check-up was just one outcome of the 2002 Health Promotion Law, an umbrella law targeting everyday lifestyle practices and behaviors as opportunities for the state to intervene to raise individuals' health consciousness and education via clinics, schools, community health centers, and companies (Manzenreiter 2012; Borovoy 2015, 2017). Nonetheless, obesity and obesity-related diseases in Japan are rising; these include dyslipidemia, diabetes, and cardiovascular disease, so-called lifestyle-related diseases. The annual health check-up and community-based weight reduction program has reported short-term successes in achieving weight reduction, but long-term success in the form of weight management remains difficult to achieve (Nakata et al. 2014; Tsukinoki et al. 2018).

Of course, the use of the word "fat" isn't always negative and damaging. Its power shifts depending on who uses it, for what purpose, and when and where and with whom. In peer fat talk, for example, having conversations around questions like "Do I look fat today?" can be a way to seek reassurance from friends, although the essential negative connotations of the word remain unchallenged (Greenhalgh 2015; Hardin 2015; Nichter 2000; SturtzSreetharan et al. 2023; Taylor 2011).

In this project, I rely on multiple meanings of fat and fatness as specifically social categories. In American English, the term "fat" shifts in power depending on who uses it, for what purposes, and when, where, and with whom. In peer fat talk, for example, having conversations around questions like "Do I look fat today?" can be a way to seek reassurance from friends or even strangers as well as a way to commiserate with peers (SturtzSreetharan et al. 2019). In Japanese, the ways in which people understand and deploy the term "futotteru" (fat) is not well understood in terms of lived experience. Certainly many terms are available for describing large body size: *himan* (obese), *metabo* (lit. metabolic syndrome, but used in place of "obese"), *futotteru* ("being fat"), *pocchari* ("chubby"), *kotteru* ("fat," Kansai regional term), and *fatto* ("fat"). But how these terms are understood, used, and perceived has yet to be investigated. Medical contexts rely on terms such as *himan* and *metabo* which are classifications of the body based on quantifiable measures (weight, height, waist and hip circumference) of appearance, not health. But the terms used by everyday Japanese people, and perhaps more importantly, the ways in which the terms are associated with fat shaming, remain underexplored.

METABOLIC SYNDROME

In Japan, metabolic syndrome (hereafter MetS) is understood as a condition that combines the measurement of visceral fat (as determined by BMI, hip and waist circumference) with high blood pressure, high blood sugar, and abnormal lipid metabolism. Each year all employed people between the ages of 40 and 74 years of age are screened for MetS as well as whether or not they use tobacco products. If an individual has one or more of the risk factors for MetS (hypertension, hyperglycaemic, and dyslipidaemia) and a waist circumference greater than 85 cm for men and 90 cm for women *or* a BMI greater than or equal to 25 then they are assigned to receive guided health interventions. People taking prescriptions medicine for these conditions are not remanded to guided intervention as it is assumed they are already addressing the underlying MetS issues (Fukuma et al. 2020). Such an intervention includes an intake interview and continuous guided support for 3–6 months; the guidance is conducted by certified professional counselors trained in nutrition, lifestyle diseases, and exercise who, themselves, are supported by physicians, public health experts, and nutritionists (Borovoy 2015, 2017; Fukuma et al. 2020, 2022). Fukuma estimates that the guided intervention program costs around $150 million per year (2022).

In FY2020, there were approximately 54.2 million people eligible for the mandatory annual health checkup but only about 53 percent (28.9 million people) received the exam (Nikkei 2023). Currently, there are roughly 9 million people (between the ages of 40 and 74) who are diagnosed with MetS in Japan, which is about 30 percent of the people who undergo the annual exam. The government has set the goals of increasing the implementation rate of specified health checkups and specified health guidance to at least 70 percent and 45 percent by FY2023, and reducing the number of persons with metabolic syndrome and those with pre-diabetes by at least 25 percent by FY2022 compared to FY2008. The Japanese government has placed employers in charge of implementation and monitoring. As such, the mandated health exam is linked directly to one's workplace/employer. It is the employer who encourages their employees to undergo the examination; in talking with many employed Japanese people, many employers try to make the process as smooth as possible. But, employees are less enamored with these efforts. For example, in talking with Sachiko (60 years old) employed at a medium-sized educational institution in the Kansai region, she told me about the large healthcare bus that comes to her workplace. The healthcare workers commandeer a few office spaces and set up a makeshift physical examination screening area. Sachiko told me that she hates entering/exiting the screening rooms in full view of her peers. Her employer allows her to go to a private clinic for the screening; the private clinic will send the results directly to her employer. The employer is tasked with both sharing the results with each employee, and alerting them to whether or not they are being recommended for guided intervention; the results are then anonymized and sent onto the appropriate national level agency. Whether one chooses a private clinic or undergoes the screening at work, the basic examination (described above) for

MetS is covered by national health insurance (a portion of which is paid for by the company).

I have been investigating the lived experience of weight in Japan since the summer of 2016, including conducting 25 in-person interviews in the summer of 2017 (SturtzSreetharan et al. 2021), followed by body image survey work in the summer of 2018 (Swami et al. 2020), and most recently research specifically about the special annual MetS exam for several months spanning April 2022–March 2023. As I talked to people about the MetS physical examination, people consistently reported that they felt anxious in the days and weeks leading up to the actual exam and that they altered their daily routines in order to feel more confidence in their ability to "pass"—that is, to not be found to have any of the markers for MetS. Thus, in what follows, I report specifically about these issues. My specific research questions are: Do people report feeling stress/anxiety in the weeks/days leading up to the exam? And, do people change their "daily behaviors" during this time? If they do alter their daily behaviors, what kinds of alterations do they make?

METHODS

Based on ethnographic interviews conducted in summer 2017 and from April to August 2022, a survey was designed to understand how people think about the special annual MetS health examination. The company, Trees Inc., located in the Kansai (western) region of Japan, was contacted to secure permission to talk with and deploy a survey (both online and in person) regarding the MetS health exam. Trees, Inc. is a company of about 300 employees the vast majority of whom are men. I initially virtually met the president of the company along with the chief operating officer and the manager of the healthcare part of their HR department (all men). After explaining the project goals, they agreed that they would send an email with a link to my participation request to all company employees. The email would come with a personal request from the company president to please consider participating. Within a week, 134 people had agreed to complete the survey questions (Table 3.3). Each of the 134 participants received a unique link to a survey. The survey instrument, delivered in Japanese, consisted of 13 questions; the first 8 questions asked about the special health exam; the final 5 questions were general demographic questions about educational level, age, assigned sex, height and weight.

Table 3.1. Questions asked of participants

1.	Have you ever undertaken the special health examination?
2.	In the days leading up to the special health examination, do you feel additional stress?
3.	Compared to a year ago, has your weight changed?
4.	In the days leading up to the special health examination, do you intentionally change your everyday routines?
5.	If you answered "yes, I change my routines" what things do you change?
6.	Has a doctor or other health professional talked to you in the past about having metabolic syndrome or lifestyle disease?
7.	Up until now, has a physician or health professional told you to lose weight?
8.	In thinking about your own body, do you ever feel judged for it?
9.	What is the highest level of education you have completed?
10.	How old are you?
11.	Are you male or female?
12.	How much do you weigh?
13.	How tall are you?

RESULTS

Of the 134 participants, 118 were men and 16 were women; the age range was 40 years old to 70 years old with an average age of 51.1 years old. Twenty-five percent (n=34) of the participants reported feeling stress that was "beyond typical" daily stress in the days leading up to the special MetS health exam. About 80 percent of the men reported feeling more than typical stress while 20 percent of women participants reported the same. While the sample size of women participants is too small to draw significant conclusions about this, almost half (7/16 or 44 percent) of the women participants reported feeling stress compared to about 22 percent of the participating men. This finding would reflect the literature which notes that women bear a heavier burden in terms of violating body size norms and appearance ideals (Brewis 2011). Twenty-six of the total number of participants reported changing their daily lifestyle behaviors in the days leading up to the special health exam. Eleven participants reported feeling more stress than is typical *and* that they change their behaviors whereas 15 participants do not report stress but still change their lifestyle behaviors. Twenty-three percent of the participants (n=31) reported feeling judged for their bodies; of these, 10 report changing their lifestyle behaviors while 19 report that they do not.

People who indicated that they change their behaviors the days and weeks prior to the special exam overwhelmingly reported that they stopped consuming alcohol, reduced their food intake, and/or increased their levels of physical activity. Food reductions included overall "meals" (*shokuji*) as well as targeted reductions such as desserts/sweets, carbohydrates, and between-meal or nighttime snacking.

Of the 31 people who reported feeling judged for their bodies, 29 of them elaborated on this felt judgment. While a few participants simply stated that they "always feel judged [for their body shape or size]" or that their body "needs improvement," other participants wrote more specific details regarding the ways that they feel judged for their body shape and size. One woman, 51-year-old Akiko, described feeling morally judged; she said that she feels like people connect her "body size and shape to an inability to manage her body [*jiko kanri*]." This idea that a larger body communicates an inability to manage the self has been found in other studies of body shame and weight in Japan (SturtzSreetharan 2021; SturtzSreetharan et al. 2021a) as well as cross-culturally. This kind of judgment, that the ability to care for oneself is called into question, reflects the sense of individual responsibility that is fundamentally tied to the biocitizen. A similar idea is captured in Kenta's reporting that because he "is short, people think he is unreliable." In this case, rather than a larger body size, Kenta feels judged for his small stature and connects it directly to how people understand his character. The free responses were read iteratively, resulting in three major themes being identified: explicit statements of body shaming, implicit acts of body shaming, and moments of self-judgments of one's own body that results in felt shame. Below I explore these themes in more detail, providing specific examples that participants noted.

Explicit Statements of Body Shaming

Some of the participants wrote about direct examples of being shamed for their body size and shape. Forty-year-old Nozomi wrote that people call him "*debu*" (fatty) or say things like "you've become fat" joking about his "expanding presence." Tetsuzo (45 years old) made a similar comment noting that people easily tell him "You've gotten fat (*futotta*)!" Shinji reported feeling "*mittomonai*" (unsightly, indecent) and self-conscious because "compared to when I was younger, I've gained 20 kgs and people say that I 'look like a different person' [*betsu jin*]." Fifty-one-year-old Asako notes that people tell her directly that she "used to be thinner" which she says is true. And, Saki explains that she feels judged for her body size and shape by her husband when he makes comments like: "you've gotten fat, haven't you!" In these examples, people are reporting their reactions to highly explicit statements that are specifically directed to them about their body shape and size. They are, in fact, being judged and experience it as felt shame.

Implicit Acts of Body Shaming

Implicit acts of body shaming were a common theme among how people described feeling that they were being judged for their body size and shape. This has been reported in other studies of felt shame around weight (Trainer et al. 2016). People report strangers staring, glancing, or "side-eyeing" them. Participants in Japan reported similar kinds of experiences and reported them as feeling judged for their body shape and size. For example, Kai (51 years old) reports that he feels judged for his style and the silhouette he casts in his clothes. Forty-nine-year-old Yuki explains that people stare directly at his belly and he feels ashamed and judged by that. Similarly, Ryusuke reports that people "stare at specific body parts," which makes him feel judged.

Moments of Self-Judgment

Moments of self-judgment can occur on purpose—checking one's style in a mirror, for example—or they can occur suddenly without preparation. In either case, negative judgments of the self due to weight is termed weight bias internalization; in short weight self-stigma (Austin et al. 2021; Durso and Latner 2008). Internalized body stigma entails feeling negatively evaluated based on a critical read of one's own body size and shape. One example of this is shared by 68-year-old Kenji, who reports that he judges his own body when he "sees a fit healthy man of the same generation [and realizes his own body is not fit]." Yusaku (57 years old) notes that when he takes a bath, he notices his body size and shape and judges himself for it. On the other hand, Junpei, 56 years old, notices his body shape and size when he is wearing clothes. He reports that his "body, especially the area around his belly, becomes really visible in summer clothing" and this embarrasses him. Likewise, Tsuneo (52 years old) reports that he is "bothered by his belly" [*Onaka no mawari ga ki ni naru*]. Clothes are also an issue for 63-year-old Taka who notes that "almost no clothing fits him [properly]" stating that finding appropriate sizes is difficult. Finally, Saburo (58 years old) simply reports that he is "fatter than he was previously" suggesting that this is something which causes him to feel judged, perhaps on a regular basis. As these comments deftly show, individuals do not simply feel judged by others—peers, family, strangers—but they experience internalized weight stigma around the appearance of their body, both their naked and clothed bodies.

DISCUSSION

In 2006 the Japanese government approved the implementation of the annual special health exam that focuses on metabolic syndrome and is accompanied by health guidance intervention for those found to have one or more indicators of the disease. The consequences of this mandatory health exam exceed the guided intervention that was originally part of the plan. This explicit health policy appears to bring anxiety to some of the people it purports to assist. In addition, people report changing their daily routines around beverages, food, and exercise in order to ensure that they will successfully "pass" the health examination. The short-term consumption changes people make include giving up alcohol, reducing food intake, and increasing physical exercise; once the special health exam is done, people resume their previous daily routines until the following year. These daily lifestyle changes are precisely in line with what the government recommended in its national Healthy Japan 21 scheme targeting various health aspects including nutrition and diet, physical activity and exercise, and tobacco and alcohol use (Nomura et al. 2022).

Most evaluations of the special health exam find that it has not reduced overall MetS diagnosis frequencies in the working population (40–74 years old); in fact, Fukuma and colleagues find evidence that among Japanese working-age people the "health guidance intervention was not associated with clinically meaningful weight loss or other cardiovascular risk factor reduction" (Fukuma 2020: 1630). In addition, while the guideline interventions may reduce outpatient visit days, it is not associated with lowering healthcare costs, hospitalizations, or medication use (Fukuma et al. 2022). If we turn to the literature that engages allostatic load, what becomes increasingly clear based on the research presented previously (SturtzSreetharan 2021; SturtzSreetharan et al. 2021a,b) is that health policies like the mandatory special health exam contributes to increased shame and stigma around body shapes and sizes that do not conform to the ideal du jour. Below I turn to exploring these thoughts more concretely based on the data already presented.

Vigilance

The participants' responses above indicate that some people view the special health exam with some trepidation. It appears to cause them to attend more carefully to their bodies, what they eat and drink, and other lifestyle behaviors. This kind of attention can be understood as "vigilance." Vigilance is a term that means attending to something carefully and constantly. It can happen for a defined duration of time or be ongoing. This idea is applied to minoritized or discriminated-against groups including people who have internalized weight bias. Vigilance refers to preparing for and remaining alert for discrimination. It is tied to poorer health (compared to those who do not need to engage in vigilance) because of the heightened physiological response necessary to maintain vigilance which is ultimately about trying to prevent stigmatizing or discriminating experiences (Lee and Hicken 2016). Negative psychosocial effects including depression, lack of sleep, increased weight, and hypertension are associated with vigilance among minoritized groups (DuBois and Juster 2022; Hicken et al. 2018; Pichardo et al. 2021), including weight stigma (Hunger et al. 2020). Important to the discussion of metabolic system, disordered eating is also associated with internalized weight stigma (Romano et al. 2021). Reflecting on the participants' reporting of greater than typical stress leading up to the special health examination, the ways that they change their daily behaviors, and the ways that they experience being judged for their body shape and size suggests that they are in a period of vigilance at least in the days leading up to the special exam and for some, constantly. Given that vigilance is known to create health problems which look like metabolic syndrome, it is important to understand the consequences of health policies that may (re)produce the very negative conditions they seek to remedy.

Biopower and Biocitizen

Biopower refers to the ways that society has control over our physical bodies (Foucault 1990). Some of this is explicit control, including educational requirements of physical education classes in elementary school, for example; or, like the Japanese government, requiring all working people between the ages of 40 and 74 to undergo a special health exam to check for metabolic syndrome. In addition, there are social norms that play a role in this process of controlling people's bodies. While the specific norms may vary across geographies and populations, it is through stigma and shame that people are encouraged to maintain their bodies in particular ways (Brewis and Wutich 2019)—especially with regard to shape and size.

A biocitizen is created through biopower when an individual assumes sole responsibility for their body and their weight (Costa 2021; Rose and Novas 2007). For some, this means doing everything they can to follow the various guidelines and social norms that their community of peers has deemed appropriate to a body: keeping fit and eating well. For others, it may mean ignoring the social stigma and pressure. The science makes clear, however, that for many the social norms and pressures to be a "good biocitizen" creates felt shame (Trainer et al., 2021); a fat body in much of the world is thought to violate widely held norms about how people should look. Japan is no exception.

The mandatory annual special health examination that screens for metabolic syndrome has brought both biopower and biocitizenry together, creating a powerful force exerted on individual Japanese people. In doing so, individuals are pressured from two sides: the national government (via their workplace) and themselves. In addition, as we have seen in the responses above, peers, family members, and strangers are also applying pressure through explicit comments and sidelong glances.

CONCLUSION

This chapter has examined working Japanese people's reports of stress and behavioral changes in the days and weeks leading up to the annual special health examination. Some people report feeling a greater level of stress than is typical during this time. People also report changing their everyday behaviors around food, alcohol, and physical activity. And, finally, many people reported feeling judged for their body size and shape. The kinds of judgments they reported included explicit statements of stigma such as that reported by Kyohei (41 years old): "[I feel judged for my body] when people say I look flabby [*buyobuyo*] and unsightly [*minikui*]." These kinds of statements come from peers, workmates, and family members. People also reported implicit acts of weight stigma including being stared at by others, sometimes in general but often specific body parts such as the belly is the target of the stigmatizing gaze. And finally, people reported judging themselves. That is, they recognize their internalized weight stigma and inflict it on themselves. Forty-two-year-old Sachi captures this when she reports matter-of-factly that "compared to the average [woman] I am fat." But it can also occur when an individual catches their reflection in a shop window or a bathroom mirror. These judgments and awareness of them reflect the vigilance that some of the people are embodying on a daily basis. It appears that the special health exam may exacerbate this vigilance. Vigilance is associated with negative physiological and psychosocial outcomes including increased hypertension, disordered eating, and depression. Each of these, in turn, often discourage an individual from engaging in physical activity and may cause people to eat more than usual (stress eating). One participant provides a particularly appropriate ending. Summing up his thoughts about the twin pressures of biopower and biocitizenry, 56-year-old Ryo says: "I wish people would leave me alone [*hotte oite hoshii*]."

REFERENCES CITED

Adams, Vincanne. 2016. *Metrics: What Counts in Global Health*. Durham, NC: Duke University Press.

Anderson-Fye, Elaine, and Alexandra Brewis, eds. 2017. *Fat Planet: Obesity, Culture & Symbolic Capital*. Albuquerque: University of New Mexico Press.

Austen, Emma, Rebecca Pearl, and Scott Griffiths. 2021. "Inconsistencies in the conceptualizations and operationalization of internalized weight stigma: A potential way forward." *Body Image* 36: iii–v.

Austin, S. Bryn. 1999. "Fat, Loathing & Public Health: The Complicity of Science in a Culture of Disordered Eating," *Culture, Medicine & Psychiatry* 23: 245–68.

Becker, Anne. 1995. *Body, Self & Society: The View from Fiji*. Philadelphia: University of Pennsylvania Press.

Borovoy, Amy. 2015. "Metabolic syndrome screening & health education: Are there lessons we can learn from Japan?" In *The Applied Anthropology of Obesity: Prevention, Intervention, & Identity,* edited by Chad Morris and Alexandra Lancey, 65–77. Lanham, MD: Lexington Books.

———. 2017. "Japan's public health paradigm: Governmentality & the containment of harmful behavior," *Medical Anthropology* 36, no. 1: 32–46.

Borovoy, Amy, and Christina Roberto. 2015. "Japanese & American public health approaches to preventing population weight gain: A role for paternalism?" *Social Science & Medicine* 143: 62–70.

Borovoy, Amy, and Li Zhang, Li. 2017. "Between biopolitical governance & care: Rethinking health, selfhood, & social welfare in East Asia," *Medical Anthropology* 36, no.1: 1–5.

Brewis, Alexandra. 2011. *Obesity: Cultural and biocultural perspectives.* New Brunswick, NJ: Rutgers University Press.

———. 2014."Stigma & the perpetuation of obesity," *Social Science & Medicine* 118: 152–58.

Brewis Alexandra, Sarah Trainer Sarah, SeungYong Han, and Amber Wutich. 2016. "Publically misfitting: Extreme weight & the everyday production & reinforcement of felt stigma," *Medical Anthropology Quarterly* 31, no. 2: 257–76.

Brewis Alexandra, and Amber Wutich. 2015. "A world of suffering? Biocultural approaches to fat stigma in the global contexts of the obesity epidemic," *Annals of Anthropological Practice* 38, no. 2: 269–83.

Brewis, Alexandra, Cindi SturtzSreetharan, and Amber Wutich. 2018. "Obesity Stigma as a Global Health Challenge," *Globalization and Health* 14:20.

Carney, Megan. 2015. *The Unending Hunger: Tracing Women & Food Insecurity Across Borders*. Berkeley: University of California Press.

Costa, Jose. 2021. "Manufacturing biocitizens: The Quantification of Bodies as a method for Incorporating a new Biomedical Ethics." In *Quantifying bodies and health. Interdisciplinary approaches* edited by J. Braga and S. Guidi, 79–87. Coleção eQVODLIBET 10, Coimbra,. https://hdl.handle.net/10362/118650.

DuBois, L. Zachary, and Robert-Paul Juster. 2022. "Lived experience and allostatic load among transmasculine people living in the United States," *Psychoneuroendocrinology* 143: 105849.

Durso, Laura, and Janet Latner. 2008. "Understanding self-directed stigma: Development of the weight bias internalization scale." *Obesity* 16 Suppl 2 S80–S86.

Fukuma, Shingo, Toshiaki Iizuka, Tatsuyoshi, Ikenoue,, and Yusuke Tsugawa, . 2020. "Association of the national health guidance intervention for obesity and cardiovascular risks with health outcomes among Japanese men," *JAMA Internal Medicine* 180 no. 12: 1630–37.

Fukuma, Shingo, Mukaigawara, Mitsuru, Iizuka, Toshiaki, and Tsugawa, Yusuke. 2022. "Impact of the national health guidance intervention for obesity and cardiovascular risks on healthcare utilization and healthcare spending in working-age Japanese cohort: regression discontinuity design," *BMJ Open* 12:e056996.

Garon, Sharon. 1997. *Molding Japanese Minds: The State in Everyday Life*. Princeton, NJ: Princeton University Press.

Garth, Hannah. 2013. "Obesity in Cuba: Memories of the Special Period & Approaches to Weight Loss Today." In *Reconstructing Obesity: The Measures of Meaning, the Meaning of Measures*, edited by Melissa McCullough and Jessica Hardin. 89–106. Oxford, NY: Berghahn.

Greenhalgh, Susan. 2015. *Fat-Talk Nation: The Human Costs of America's War on Fat*. Ithaca, NY: Cornell University Press.

Hardin, Jessica. 2015. "Christianity, Fat Talk, and Samoan Pastors: Rethinking the Fat-Positive-Fat-Stigma Framework," *Fat Studies* 4 no. 2: 178–96. https://doi.org/10.1080/21604851.2015.1015924.

Hardin, Jessica, Amy McLennan, and Alexandra Brewis. 2018. "Body size, body norms & some unintended consequences of obesity intervention in the Pacific Islands." *Annals of Human Biology* 45 no. 3: 285–94.

Hicken, Margaret, Hedwig Lee, and Anna Hing. 2018. "The weight of racism: Vigilance and racial inequalities in weight-related measures," *Social Science and Medicine*, 199: 157–166. https://doi.org/10.1016/j.socscimed.2017.03.058.

Himmelstein, Mary, Rebecca Puhl, and Diane Quinn. 2018. "Weight stigma in men: What, when, and by whom?" *Obesity* 26, no. 6: 968–76.

Hunger, Jeffrey, and Brenda Major. 2015. "Weight stigma mediates the association between BMI and self-reported health." *Health Psychology* 34, no. 2, 172–75. https://doi.org/10.1037/hea0000106.

Hunger, Jeffrey, Dodd, Dorian, and April Smith. 2020. "Weight discrimination, anticipated weight stigma, and disordered eating," *Eating Behaviors* 37: Article 101383. https://doi.org/10.1016/j.eatbeh.2020.101383.

Jutel, Annemarie. 2006. "The Emergence of Overweight as a Disease Entity: Measuring up Normality," *Social Science & Medicine* 63: 2268–76.

LeBesco, Kathleen. 2011. "Neoliberalism, public health, & the moral perils of fatness," *Critical Public Health* 21, no. 2: 153–64.

Lee, Hedwig, and Margaret Hicken. 2016. "Death by a thousand cuts: The health implications of black respectability politics," *Souls* 18, no. 2–4: 421–45. https://doi.org/10.1080/10999949.2016.1230828.

Lewis, Catherine. 1995. *Educating Hearts & Minds: Reflections on Japanese Preschool & Elementary Education.* Cambridge: Cambridge University Press.

Manzenreiter, Wolfram. 2012. "Monitoring health & the body: Anthropometry, life-style risks, & the Japanese obesity crisis," *Journal of Japanese Studies* 38, no. 1: 55–84.

McCullough, Melissa, and Jessica Hardin, eds. 2013. *Reconstructing Obesity Research: The Measures of Meaning, the Meaning of Measures*. Oxford, NY: Berghahn.

Melby, Melissa, and Wakako Takeda. 2014. "Lifestyle constraints, not inadequate nutrition education, cause gap between breakfast ideals & realities among Japanese in Tokyo," *Appetite* 72, no. 1: 37–49.

Monaghan, Lee 2005. "Big handsome men, bears, and others: Virtual constructions of 'fat male embodiment,'" *Body & Society* 11, no. 2: 81–111.

———. 2007. "Body Mass Index, masculinities and moral worth: Men's critical understandings of 'appropriate' weight-for-height." *The Sociology of Health & Illness*, 29, no. 4: 584–609.

——— 2008. *Men and the War on Obesity: A Sociological Study*. Routledge Press,.

Monaghan, Lee, Rachel Colls, and Bethan Evans. 2013. "Obesity Discourse & Fat Politics: Research, Critique & Interventions," *Critical Public Health* 23, no. 3: 249–62.

Nakata Yoshio, Masafumi Okada, Koichi Hashimoto, and Yoshinori Harada 2014. "Weight loss maintenance for 2 years after a 6-month randomized controlled trial comparing education-only & group-based support in Japanese adults," *Obesity Facts* 7, no. 6: 376–87.

Nichter, Mimi. 2000. *Fat Talk*: *What Girls and Their Parents Say about Dieting*. Cambridge, MA: Harvard University Press.

Nikkei, "Niigata and Gifu, both with low metabolic syndrome rates, benefit from exercise promotion apps and low-sodium diets: Regional revitalization through data." *Nihon Keizai Shimbun*. Accessed Aug 8, 2023. https://www.nikkei.com/article/DGXZQOCC143W30U3A610C2000000/.

Nomura, Shuhei, Haruka Sakamoto, Cyrus Ghaznavi, and Manami Inoue. 2022. "Toward a third term of Health Japan 21—implications from the rise in non-communicable disease burden and highly preventable risk factors." *The Lancet Regional Health—Western Pacific* 21: 100377.

Pichardo, Catherine, Kristine Molina, Carlos Rosas, Marbella Uriostegui, and Lisa Sanchez-Johnsen. 2021. "Racial discrimination and depressive symptoms among Latina/o college students: The role of racism-related vigilance and sleep," *Race and Social Problems* 13, no. 2: 86–101. https://doi.org/10.1007/s12552-020-09304-1.

Popenoe, Rebecca. 2003. *Feeding Desire: Fatness, Beauty & Sexuality Among a Saharan People*. London: Routledge.

Popkin, Barry, and Penny Gordon-Larsen. 2004. "The Nutrition Transition: Worldwide Obesity Dynamics & Their Determinants." *International Journal of Obesity* 28: 2–9.

Popkin, Barry, Linda Adair, Linda, Shu Wen Ng. 2012. "Global Nutrition Transition & the Pandemic of Obesity in Developing Countries." *Nutrition Reviews* 70, no. 1: 3–21.

Puhl, Rebecca, and Kelly Brownell. 2006. "Confronting & coping with weight stigma: an investigation of overweight & obese adults," *Obesity* 14: 1802–15.

Puhl, Rebecca, and Chelsea Heuer. 2009. "The stigma of obesity: A review & update," *Obesity* 17: 941–64.

Puhl Rebecca, Joerg Luedicke, and Jamie Lee Peterson. 2013. "Public reactions to obesity-related health campaigns: A randomized controlled trial," *American Journal of Preventative Medicine* 45, no. 1: 36–48.

Romano, Kelly, Kristin Heron, James Henson. 2021. "Examining associations among weight stigma, weight bias internalization, body dissatisfaction, and eating disorder symptoms: Does weight status matter?" *Body Image* 37: 38–49. https://doi.org/10.1016/j.bodyim.2021.01.006.

Rose, Nikolas, and Carlos Novas. 2007. "Biological citizenship." In *Global Assemblages: Technology, Politics, and Ethics as Anthropological Problems*, edited by Aiwha Ong and Stephen Collier, 439–63. Blackwell Publishing.

Sanabria, Emilia, and Emily Yates-Doerr. 2015. "Alimentary uncertainties: From contest evidence to policy," *BioSocieties* 10: 117–24.

Scagliusi, Fernanda, Mariana Ulian, Bruno Gualano, Odilon Roble, Ramiro Unsain, Maria Carriero, Priscila de Morais Sato, Cindi SturtzSreetharan, Alexandra Brewis, and Amber Wutich. 2020. "'Before I saw a gas canister, now I see a person': Post-intervention qualitative differences in body acceptance and response to weight stigma in everyday lives among Brazilian 'gorda' women living with obesity." *Human Organization* 79, no. 3: 176–91. https://doi.org/10.17730/1938-3525-79.3.176.

Sobo, Elise. 1994. "The Sweetness of Fat: Health, Procreation, & Sociability in Rural Jamaica." In *Many Mirrors: Body Image & Social Relations*, edited by Nicole Sault, 133–53. Rutgers University Press.

SturtzSreetharan, Cindi, Sarah Trainer, Amber Wutich, and Alexandra Brewis. 2018. "Moral Biocitizenship: Discursively managing food and the body after Bariatric Surgery." *Journal of Linguistic Anthropology* 28, no. 2: 221–40.

SturtzSreetharan, Cindi, Gina Agostini, Amber Wutich, Alexandra Brewis, Charlayne Mitchell, Olivia Rines, and Brittany Romanello. 2019. " 'I need to lose some weight:' Masculinity and body image as negotiated through fat talk," *Psychology of Men and Masculinity* 21, no. 1: 148–61.

SturtzSreetharan, Cindi, and Alexandra Brewis. 2019. "Rice, men, and other everyday anxieties: Navigating obesogenic urban food environments in Osaka, Japan," In *Handbook of Global Urban Health* edited by Igor Vojnovic, Amber Pearson, Asiki Gershim, Geoffrey Deverteuil, and Adriana Allen, 545–64. Routledge.

SturtzSreetharan, Cindi. 2021. "'My body doesn't hinder me, so I'm satisfied': Enacting a Japanese life through lingual life histories," *Journal of Anthropological Research* 77, no. 1: 67–82.

SturtzSreetharan, Cindi, Alexandra Brewis, Jessica Hardin, Sarah Trainer, and Amber Wutich. 2021a. *Fat in Four Cultures: A global ethnography of weight*. University of Toronto Press.

SturtzSreetharan, Cindi, Sarah Trainer, and Alexandra Brewis. 2021b. "The Harm Inflicted by Polite Concern: Language, Fat, and Stigma," *Culture, Medicine, and Psychiatry* 46, no. 4: 683–709 DOI: 10.1007/s11013-021-09742-5.

SturtzSreetharan, Cindi, Monet Ghorbani, Amber Wutich, and Alexandra Brewis. 2023. "Deny, Reassure, and Deflect: Evidence and Implications of Forms and Norms of Fat Talk," *Cross Cultural Research.*

Swami, Viren, Ulrich Tran, David Barron, Reza Afhami, Annie Aimé, Carlos Almenara, Nursel Dal, et al. 2020. "The breast size satisfaction survey (BSSS): Breast size dissatisfaction and its antecedents and outcomes in women from 40 nations," *Body Image* 32: 199–217. https://doi.org/10.1016/j.bodyim.2020.01.006.

Taylor, John. 2010. "Janus and the Siren's Call: Kave and the Articulation of Gender and Modernity in Vanuatu. " *Journal of Royal Anthropological Institute* 16: 279–96.

Taylor, Nicole L. 2011 "Negotiating Popular Obesity Discourses in Adolescence," *Food, Culture & Society* 14, no. 4: 587–606. https://doi.org/10.2752/175174411X13046092851433.

Tomiyama, A. Janet. 2014. "Weight stigma is stressful. A review of evidence for the cyclic obesity/weight-based stigma model." *Appetite* 82: 8–15. https://doi.org/10.1016/j.appet.2014.06.108.

Tomiyama, A. Janet, Deborah Carr, Ellen Granberg, Brenda Major, Eric Robinson, Angelina Sutin, and Alexandra Brewis. 2018 "How and why weight stigma drives the obesity 'epidemic' and harms health," *BMC Medicine* 16, no. 1: Article 123. https://doi.org/10.1186/s12916-018-1116-5.

Trainer, Sarah, Alexandra Brewis, Amber Wutich, Liza Kurtz, and Monet Niesluchowski. 2016. "The fat self in virtual communities: Success & failure in weight-loss blogging." *Current Anthropology* 57, no. 4: 523–28.

Trainer, Sarah, Alexandra Brewis, and Amber Wutich. 2021. *Extreme Weight Loss: Life Before and After Bariatric Surgery*. New York: New York University Press.

Trainer, Sarah, Cindi SturtzSreetharan, Amber Wutich, Alexandra Brewis, and Jessica Hardin. 2022. "Fat is all my fault: Globalized metathemes of body self-blame." *MAQ* 36, no. 1:5–26 DOI: 10.1111/maq.12687.

Tsukinoki, Rumi, Tomonori Okamura, Nagako Okuda, Aya Kadota, Yoshitaka Murakami, Masahiko Yanagita, Naomi Miyamatsu, et al. 2018. "One-year weight loss maintenance outcomes following a worksite-based weight reduction program among Japanese men with cardiovascular risk factors." *Journal of Occupational Health* 61, no. 2: 189–96.

Ulian, Mariana, Ramiro Unsain, Ruth Franco, Marco Aurélio Santo, Alexandra Brewis, Sarah Trainer, Cindi SturtzSreetharan, Amber Wutich, Bruno Gualano, and Fernanda Baeza Scagliusi. 2023. "Weight stigma after bariatric surgery: A qualitative study with Brazilian women." *PLoSOne* 18, no. 7:e0287822.

Westermann, Stefan, Rief Winfried, Frank Euteneuer, and Sebastian Kohlmann. 2015. "Social exclusion & shame in obesity." *Eating Behaviors* 17: 74–76.

Yates-Doerr, Emily. 2015. *The Weight of Obesity: Hunger & Global Health in Postwar Guatemala*. Berkeley: University of California Press.

Chapter 4

Who Gets PrEPped? Negotiating Barriers to Agency for HIV Prevention

Stacy W. Smallwood and Dorcas Ama Adom

Human immunodeficiency virus (HIV) remains a significant health issue across the world, with approximately 39 million people living with HIV and 1.3 million new HIV infections globally (UNAIDS 2023). At the end of 2021, about 1.2 million people were estimated to be living with HIV, with approximately 36,000 new diagnoses that year (CDC 2022). Significant HIV disparities exist in the United States, as there are certain groups that are disproportionately represented in new diagnoses and people living with HIV (CDC 2023). For example, men who have sex with men, African American and Hispanic/Latino people, and people living in the South account for a disproportionate number of people living with HIV (CDC 2023). Therefore, a health equity lens is critical to preventing new infections and helping people living with HIV achieve viral suppression.

In the four decades since the HIV/AIDS epidemic was first identified in the United States, multiple biomedical and behavioral interventions, such as HIV testing, antiretroviral therapies (ART), and condom use have reduced the number of new infections and improved the health and quality of life for people living with HIV (Fauci and Lane 2020). However, the need for additional types of prevention intervention persists. In the absence of a federally approved vaccine for HIV, one watershed moment for HIV prevention was the introduction of pre-exposure prophylaxis (PrEP) as a biomedical strategy for people who are HIV-negative. Approved by the Food and Drug Administration in 2012, PrEP use has been determined to be up to 99 percent effective in preventing HIV acquisition (Fauci and Lane 2020; Louisiana

Health Hub, 2023; NIH 2021). PrEP has been identified as a key component in the U.S. Department of Health and Human Services' "Ending the HIV Epidemic: A Plan for the United States" (EHE) initiative, with the goals of reducing new HIV infections in the United States by 90 percent by the year 2030 (Fauci et al. 2019).

Despite the promising evidence supporting its use, PrEP uptake has been slow and uneven, particularly among individuals in demographic groups who are disproportionately affected by the HIV epidemic and/or who live in regions highly impacted by the epidemic (Siegler et al. 2018; Sullivan et al. 2019; Ming et al. 2020). As communities and public health professionals seek to both understand factors associated with PrEP uptake and develop strategies to increase uptake, it is important to examine the role of agency in the negotiation of PrEP use. The following chapter will interrogate the multifaceted ways in which agency impacts PrEP use, and provide suggestions for future research and practice.

WHAT IS PREP?

The Centers for Disease Control and Prevention define PrEP as a medication that lessens the risk of contracting HIV through sexual intercourse or drug injection (CDC 2023; Sewell et al. 2021). Initially, PrEP was approved for use as a once-daily oral pill (Biello et al. 2017; NIH 2021). In 2012, after clinical trials, the FDA approved the use of a fixed dose combination of emtricitabine (FTC) and tenofovir disoproxil fumarate (TDF) in combination with safer sex practices for HIV-negative individuals who are at high risk of acquiring HIV (CDC 2014; Dubov et al. 2018). In 2019, a new pharmaceutical combination of emtricitabine (FTC) and tenofovir alafenimide (TAF) was approved for use as PrEP, but only for men and transgender women (Hiv 2019; Sullivan et al. 2018). In 2021, the FDA approved the use of a cabotegravir injectable as a new PrEP option that would not require a daily oral pill, instead being administered once every two months (Commissioner 2021).

Parallel to the early discovery of PrEP as a preventative tool, some biomedical researchers described PrEP as a way of medicalization or argued that there was a foreseeable HIV drug resistance while social science researchers also examined the ways in which PrEP could be integrated into safer sex ethics (Brisson, Ravitsky, and Williams-Jones 2019). Over a period of time, social scientists began to investigate the social and cultural factors influencing its conception, implementation, and use, with the goal to better understand how it can bring about social and psychological transformation within LGBT communities (Brisson, Ravitsky, and Williams-Jones 2019; Spieldenner 2016). For example, social scientists have over the years conducted research on the impact of PrEP on anxiety and depression among gay, bisexual and other men who have sex with men. Recently, PrEP has gained wide recognition as a crucial technique for halting the HIV epidemic and a critical component of integrated HIV prevention strategies (Shrestha and Copenhaver 2018; Spieldenner 2016) as it gives individuals agency over their HIV vulnerability, relieving people who might otherwise fret about whether their partners will use a condom, receive antiretroviral therapy, or truthfully reveal their HIV status. Agency, in this context, is defined as the capacity and autonomy to act on an individual's behalf (Grant and Koester 2016).

IN THE UNITED STATES, WHAT ARE THE DISPARITIES BETWEEN THOSE WHO COULD BENEFIT FROM PREP USE VS. THOSE WHO ARE ACTUALLY USING/BEING PRESCRIBED PREP?

Despite evidence that declines in new HIV infections are strongest where PrEP has been administered, PrEP implementation is slow, especially among marginalized communities with disproportionate HIV burden, including racial, ethnic, and sexual minority groups (Barreras, Linnemayr, and MacCarthy 2019; Dubov et al. 2018; Mayer, Agwu, and Malebranche 2020; Nicol, Adams, and Kashuba 2013; Ming et al. 2020; Sewell et al. 2021). Although some of the factors related to lower PrEP uptake are individual in nature (e.g., awareness, knowledge), many of them are related to social and systemic barriers that constrain PrEP access and acceptability among these populations (Mayer, Agwu, and Malebranche 2020).

Additional demographic characteristics provide more complex, intersectional views of HIV vulnerability in the United States. The South, which accounted for 38 percent of the US population, carried approximately 52 percent of the burden of new HIV infections in 2021 (CDC 2023; Eaton et al. 2017; Keen and Bavinton 2020; Sullivan et al. 2019). Nationwide, Black women comprised 54 percent of new HIV diagnoses in 2019 (CDC 2022). Women's risk for HIV is generally viewed as a result of their propensity to exploitation, violence, and feudal moralities (Cairns, Race, and Goicochea 2016; Bradley et al. 2019; Hartmann and Lanham 2019). Relatedly, HIV incidence has been chronically high among Black MSM, who accounted for 26 percent of new HIV infections in 2021 (Brooks et al. 2020; Campbell et al. 2022; CDC 2023). Since 2011, new diagnoses have surged yearly among MSM aged 25–34 years (CDC 2016; Brooks et al. 2020; Sullivan et al. 2019) and the prevalence of HIV diagnoses among Black individuals has risen over time, from 29 percent in 1981 to 41 percent in 2019, when Black people made up 17 percent and 14 percent of the US population, respectively, according to HIV surveillance data reported by Bosh et al. (2019). Black transgender women were overrepresented among incident HIV diagnoses, representing 46 percent of all diagnoses among transgender women and Black transgender men comprising 41 percent of all diagnoses among transgender men (Campbell et al. 2023; CDC 2023).

Given these disparities in HIV vulnerability, one might view PrEP as a "great equalizer" in addressing the epidemic. However, evidence suggests that many individuals who could benefit from PrEP use are not using it (Kimatini et al. 2023; Quinn, Bowleg and Dickson-Gomez 2019). A 2015 study report by the CDC indicated that around 1.2 million persons living in the United States had PrEP indications; however, just 49,158 people, that is 4 percent of the population, were using PrEP (Dubov et al. 2018; Ming et al. 2020). Several studies that have examined barriers to PrEP initiation and adherence among MSM have been limited to certain categories of vulnerable groups (Biello et al. 2017; Brooks et al. 2019; Brooks et al. 2020; Eaton et al. 2017) For example, only 9 percent (42,372) of the almost 469,000 Black adults with an indication for PrEP usage had a prescription (CDC 2019).

PrEP use may also be inadequate in persons who inject drugs (PWID) (Edelman et al. 2017). A survey of primary care physicians found that more than one-quarter were unwilling to prescribe PrEP to PWID, despite the fact that certain PWID are at high risk of HIV acquisition (Edelman et al. 2017; Storholm et al. 2021; Turner et al. 2018; Ming et al. 2020; NIH 2021). Cisgender women at risk of HIV also used PrEP at a low rate (McMahan et al. 2019; Sullivan et al. 2018). Based on commercial US pharmacy statistics, the estimated annual percentage change (EAPC) for women initiating PrEP increased by 5 percent between 2012 and 2017, whereas it increased by 68 percent for males (Siegler et al. 2018). This further illustrates a disparity in PrEP use for women juxtaposed to their need, since women accounted for more than a quarter of new HIV infections in 2016 (Sullivan et al. 2018).

Research suggests that knowledge and awareness of PrEP, perception of HIV risk, stigma from healthcare providers or family, partners and friends, victimization, homelessness, unequal power dynamics, distrust of healthcare providers and systems, access and costs of PrEP, and concerns about PrEP side effects interactions are among the many structural, social, clinical, and behavioral barriers (Biello et al. 2017; Calabrese and Underhill 2015; Calabrese et al. 2018; Dubov et al. 2018; Grant and Koester 2016; Mayer, Agwu, and Malebranche 2020; McNulty et al. 2022).

Age may also play a significant role in PrEP adoption. Young people at risk for HIV acquisition had lower levels of PrEP usage compared to their need (Marks et al. 2017). According to (Siegler et al. 2018), in a 2017 prescription-level data study, PrEP usage in individuals under the age of 24 was 15.2 per 100,000 people, with a PrEP-to-need ratio (PnR; the ratio of PrEP users to new HIV diagnoses) of 0.9. In comparison, PrEP use was 61.5 per 100,000 people aged 24–35. Moreso, geography may play a role in the disparities in PrEP use rates (Huang et al. 2018) For example, despite the fact that men and women in the South accounted for 52 percent of US HIV infections in 2017, only 27 percent of PrEP users were from the southern part of the United States (CDC 2022; Sullivan et al. 2019).

Given the disparities in PrEP prescription and uptake among vulnerable populations, particularly minoritized communities, it is important to interrogate the role of agency in PrEP use as a way to unsettle commonly held narratives. Many public health interventions are developed with the expectation that various publics will automatically gravitate toward them based on novelty or the support of an authoritative, often governmental, voice. However, such simplistic, reductive approaches to public health promotion, including PrEP, can lead to underuse. In other words, public health innovation does not guarantee diffusion; just because we "build it" does not guarantee that they will "come," regardless of the presence or understanding of epidemiological evidence. Diverse communities, based on their minoritized social locations, may not have the same space to exercise full agency compared to their more normative counterparts. Therefore, examining and incorporating the role of agency in PrEP promotion can be a powerful way to support uptake and also value the lived experiences of those who are most vulnerable to HIV acquisition.

WHAT PREVIOUS RESEARCH HAS ADDRESSED THE ROLE OF AGENCY OR CONTROL IN PREP USE/UPTAKE?

Much of the extant research related to PrEP agency has been in the realm of PrEP stigma, which can be defined as the negative social connotations associated with those who engage in PrEP use (Calabrese and Underhill 2015; Calabrese 2020). Calabrese (2020) and Earnshaw and Chaudoir (2009) state that stigma can be enacted, projected, or internalized. Enacted stigma refers to overt acts of discrimination, such as social rejection, and violence; anticipated stigma is the expectation or belief that future acts of prejudice and discrimination will occur; and internalized stigma is the degree to which an individual endorses negative perceptions or feelings about themselves (Earnshaw and Chaudoir 2009). PrEP stigma can span all of these manifestations, yet remains rooted in notions of power and social hierarchy, such that people who use PrEP may be mislabeled, devalued, and discriminated against, and those perceptions can be internalized (Calabrese and Underhill 2015; Calabrese 2020). PrEP stigma can be characterized in multiple ways, including: fear of being misidentified as a person living with HIV; concerns about the perceptions of family and friends; associations with behaviors deemed socially unacceptable; or perceptions that a PrEP use serves as an enabler for individuals to engage in "risky" sexual behaviors, such as condomless sex or sex with multiple partners (Brooks et al. 2019; Golub 2018; Mayer, Agwu, and Malebranche 2020). Thus, PrEP stigma has been identified as a factor associated with PrEP hesitancy and discontinuation (Brooks et al. 2019; Golub 2018; Mayer, Agwu, and Malbranche 2020). Yet, research by Keene et al. (2021) indicated that gay, bisexual and same-gender-loving individuals who report stronger familial support have higher self-esteem and progress in their gender confirmation. Although there is limited research, these findings convey that family support may play an important role in facilitating PrEP uptake among at-risk Black and Latino transgender women and enhancing their overall mental and emotional well-being (Brooks et al. 2019). Therefore, PrEP should be viewed as more than just a treatment; it should be a tool for facilitating agency (Cairns, Race, and Goicochea 2016).

PrEP stigma is not limited to social experiences; it also manifests itself in clinical settings. Specifically, the perceptions of medical providers can circumscribe PrEP access, even for those who are clinically indicated for PrEP. Physicians often serve as the gateway to PrEP access; however, research has shown that lower levels of PrEP knowledge among providers are associated with lower rates of PrEP prescription, as well as decreased intent to prescribe PrEP in the future (Blumenthal et al. 2015; Castel et al. 2015; Pinto et al. 2018; Storholm et al. 2021). In addition to knowledge deficits among providers, subjective perceptions about individuals' PrEP eligibility and appropriateness persist. For example, providers may be less likely to prescribe PrEP if they perceive that their patients do not meet their definitions of being "at risk," such as being married or in long-term relationships. Finally, the patient-provider relationship must be interrogated as a potential barrier to agency, as the power differential between clinicians and patients could also discourage potential PrEP-indicated individuals from gaining access to PrEP.

WHAT ARE THE GAPS IN THE LITERATURE REGARDING AGENCY AND PREP FOR GAY, BISEXUAL, AND SAME-GENDER-LOVING MEN OF COLOR AND HETEROSEXUAL WOMEN OF COLOR?

Several studies have revealed that vulnerabilities exist in groups such as: gay, bisexual, and other MSM; social and individualized factors such as mental illnesses, occurrences of violence based on gender or transphobia, poverty, imprisonment, and a higher prevalence of sex work all contribute to elevated

HIV risk profile (CDC 2023; Grant and Koester 2016; McNulty et al. 2022; Keen and Bavinton 2020). Disparities in oral PrEP use persist despite its widespread acceptance and robust studies that support its safety, efficacy and significant promise to bend the HIV curve in areas at highest risk for HIV (Campbell et al. 2022). Over the years, PrEP research pertaining to HIV among gay, bisexual, PWID and same-gender-loving individuals have focused on three well-known areas: use and intake rates, side effects and efficacy, and how individuals modify their behavior in accordance to their perceived risk level (Alcantar Heredia and Goldklank 2021). Another angle of PrEP activism in the United States aims to increase public awareness of the rising rates of new HIV infections among black and Latinx people, prioritize the issue of health access and treatment for people regardless of their social standing or financial resources, and provide a non-stigmatizing, empowering, and relatable voice to the populations currently most impacted by the epidemic (Barreras, Linnemayr, and MacCarthy 2019; Biello et al. 2017; Calabrese et al. 2018; Dehlin et al. 2019).

Unfortunately, the concept of agency, particularly in light of PrEP usage, has received little attention in the lives of gay, bisexual, and same-gender-loving men of color and heterosexual women of color. One of the numerous health and social movements that have flourished through organization and agitation is the activism surrounding PrEP in the face of pharmaceutical and societal apathy. While there is current research on PrEP use, adherence, and hurdles, there is a relative lack of studies that look at agency and how it affects PrEP decision-making and use in these specific groups (Cairns, Race, and Goicochea 2016; Dehlin et al. 2019). As such, Dehlin et al. (2019) suggest that diseases like HIV or AIDS necessitate modern public health solutions focused on health equity in order to minimize the growing disparities among various racial societies in the United States.

An international lens can also help us to understand the role of agency in PrEP use domestically. Research by (Cairns, Race, and Goicochea 2016) found that during the analysis of what could have been a setback in the PrEP trials in Cambodia and Cameroon, USAID and the Global Campaign for Microbicides deduced that whereas participants were contacted about the PrEP trials, they were not involved in the planning. Gilead, the only pharmaceutical company that was approved by the FDA to manufacture and distribute PrEP initially, stated that PrEP was not an avenue for profits, hence it did not market the product on a commercial basis (Dehlin et al. 2019). This regrettable decision has had an impact on individuals who genuinely need it in a number of ways.

As qualitative research has shown, collaboration is an effective indicator for adherence, and in order to achieve health equity, one must consider how individual outcomes and structural oppressions contribute to the worsening health disparities in American communities affected by HIV/AIDS (Bradley et al. 2019; Dehlin et al. 2019). To validate these research findings, it is not surprising that interventions developed by state-led and pharmaceutical alliances that are remote from these areas run the danger of being irrelevant or insulting without input from local community people affected by the epidemic of HIV (Dehlin et al. 2019).

Also, there are gaps in the evidence about the cultural and societal elements that determine agency and PrEP usage in these communities. Stigma, discrimination, cultural norms, community support, and healthcare access may have differing effects on agency for same-gender-loving men of color, gay, bisexual and heterosexual women of color (Bernays et al. 2021; Brooks et al. 2020; Alcantar Heredia and Goldklank 2021; Mayer, Agwu, and Malebranche 2020). Thus, there is a clear need to look more closely at the variables that influence PrEP use when comparing the overall burden of HIV among Black persons to rates of PrEP coverage.

HOW CAN AGENCY BE MAXIMIZED TO FACILITATE PREP UPTAKE AMONG THESE POPULATIONS?

Based on previous studies in this area, one may be led to think of agency as a primarily individual-level factor associated with PrEP uptake. However, a social ecological approach (Golden et al. 2015; McLeroy et al. 1988) suggests that agency should be considered across multiple levels of influence. The consideration of multilevel approaches can lead to more comprehensive, effective interventions to facilitate and increase PrEP uptake (Irungu, Khoza and Velloza 2021; Pinto et al. 2018). As noted previously, individual agency for PrEP use is hindered by the presence of multiple stigmas that members of marginalized communities vulnerable to HIV acquisition often face—stigmas related to their social identities, including race, gender identity, class, and sexuality, among others. In order for members of these communities to feel more empowered to use PrEP as an HIV prevention tool, work must be done to dismantle the many intersectional prejudices, stereotypes, and biases that malign them within society. For example, PrEP stigma is strongly associated with notions of hypersexuality, promiscuity, and irresponsibility that are commonly associated with immorality (Calabrese 2020). For Black people in the United States, these stigmas are rooted in centuries-old racist beliefs that have been deployed to justify state-sanctioned discrimination, segregation, and violence. To decrease PrEP stigma at the individual and interpersonal levels, the persisting stigmas of racism, misogyny, classism, and homophobia must be systematically combated.

PrEP agency is not only based on perceptions and stereotypes; access to PrEP also remains a fundamental barrier to agency. Although efforts to increase PrEP availability are underway through governmental and nonprofit public health initiatives, significant barriers in the healthcare system remain. Increasing the number and location of pathways to PrEP, such as pharmacists' ability to prescribe PrEP as opposed to requiring a physician's prescription, can support PrEP access in ways that are not as heavily stigmatized. However, that access must also be accompanied by increased low- or no-cost access to routine HIV testing and lab screening to ensure proper liver and kidney function.

Finally, in addition to combating stigma and increasing access, community engagement should be a central pillar of any approach to foster and support PrEP agency. Far too often, community voice has been ignored or undervalued when developing health interventions, whether biomedical or behavioral. In the case of PrEP, the communities and populations most affected by HIV should be centered in the development of campaigns, programs, and other initiatives designed to increase uptake. An example of a community-led initiative is PrEP in Black America (PIBA), which is composed of Black community advocates, health practitioners, and scholars from across the United States (Campbell et al. 2023). PIBA has held community summits in locations where Black people have been significantly affected by the HIV epidemic, including cities like Atlanta and New Orleans, to directly engage local communities in dialogue about how best to facilitate PrEP access for Black people in their local contexts. In 2023, PIBA produced a report detailing a road map for increasing PrEP uptake in Black communities (Campbell et al. 2023). The group also engages government officials and policymakers at local, state, and federal levels to ensure that future policy proposals are informed by the perspectives and lived experiences of Black community members from across the nation. Future efforts to promote PrEP uptake in vulnerable communities should consider how to foster initiatives like PIBA that prioritize and amplify community voice.

Although PrEP has been considered a "game changer" in efforts to end the HIV epidemic, many Black communities have had their agency for PrEP use constrained by structures and social stigmas. Comprehensive, multilevel approaches are needed to ensure that Black communities, in particular, have the confidence, ability, and access to be in control of their sexual health.

REFERENCES CITED

Alcantar Heredia, Jorge L., and Shelly Goldklank. 2021. "The Relevance of Pre-Exposure Prophylaxis in Gay Men's Lives and Their Motivations to Use It: A

Qualitative Study." *BMC Public Health* 21, no. 1 (December): 1829. https://doi.org/10.1186/s12889-021-11863-w.

Barreras, J. L., S. L. Linnemayr, and S. MacCarthy. 2019. "'We Have a Stronger Survival Mode': Exploring Knowledge Gaps and Culturally Sensitive Messaging of PrEP among Latino Men Who Have Sex with Men and Latina Transgender Women in Los Angeles, CA." *AIDS Care* 31, no. 10 (October): 1221–27. https://doi.org/10.1080/09540121.2019.1601669.

Bernays, Sarah, Adam Bourne, Susan Kippax, Peter Aggleton, and Richard Parker. 2021. "Remaking HIV Prevention: The Promise of TasP, U=U and PrEP." In *Remaking HIV Prevention in the 21st Century: The Promise of TasP, U=U and PrEP*, edited by Sarah Bernays, Adam Bourne, Susan Kippax, Peter Aggleton, and Richard Parker, 1–18. Social Aspects of HIV. Cham: Springer International Publishing. https://doi.org/10.1007/978-3-030-69819-5_1.

Biello, Katie B., Catherine E. Oldenburg, Jennifer A. Mitty, Elizabeth F. Closson, Kenneth H. Mayer, Steven A. Safren, and Matthew J. Mimiaga. 2017. "The 'Safe Sex' Conundrum: Anticipated Stigma From Sexual Partners as a Barrier to PrEP Use Among Substance Using MSM Engaging in Transactional Sex." *AIDS and Behavior* 21, no. 1 (January): 300–306. https://doi.org/10.1007/s10461-016-1466-y.

Blumenthal, Jill, Sonia Jain, Douglas Krakower, Xiaoying Sun, Jason Young, Kenneth Mayer, Richard Haubrich, and The CCTG 598 Team. 2015. "Knowledge Is Power! Increased Provider Knowledge Scores Regarding Pre-Exposure Prophylaxis (PrEP) Are Associated with Higher Rates of PrEP Prescription and Future Intent to Prescribe PrEP." *AIDS and Behavior* 19, no. 5 (May): 802–10. https://doi.org/10.1007/s10461-015-0996-z.

Bosh, Karin A., Irene Hall, Laura Eastham, Demetre C. Daskalakis, and Jonathan H. Mermin. "Estimated Annual Number of HIV Infections—United States, 1981–2019." *MMWR. Morbidity and Mortality Weekly Report* 70 (2021). https://doi.org/10.15585/mmwr.mm7022a1.

Bradley, Erin, Kaitlin Forsberg, Joshua E. Betts, Julia B. DeLuca, Emiko Kamitani, Sarah E. Porter, Theresa Ann Sipe, and Karen W. Hoover. 2019. "Factors Affecting Pre-Exposure Prophylaxis Implementation for Women in the United States: A Systematic Review." *Journal of Women's Health* 28, no. 9 (September): 1272–85. https://doi.org/10.1089/jwh.2018.7353.

Brisson, Julien, Vardit Ravitsky, and Bryn Williams-Jones. 2019. "Towards an Integration of PrEP into a Safe Sex Ethics Framework for Men Who Have Sex with Men." *Public Health Ethics* 12, no. 1 (April): 54–63. https://doi.org/10.1093/phe/phy018.

Brooks, Ronald A., Amanda Landrian, Omar Nieto, and Anne Fehrenbacher. 2019. "Experiences of Anticipated and Enacted Pre-Exposure Prophylaxis (PrEP) Stigma Among Latino MSM in Los Angeles." *AIDS and Behavior* 23, no. 7 (July): 1964–73. https://doi.org/10.1007/s10461-019-02397-9.

Brooks, Ronald A., Omar Nieto, Amanda Landrian, Anne Fehrenbacher, and Alejandra Cabral. 2020. "Experiences of Pre-Exposure Prophylaxis (PrEP)–Related Stigma among Black MSM PrEP Users in Los Angeles." *Journal of Urban Health* 97, no. 5 (October): 679–91. https://doi.org/10.1007/s11524-019-00371-3.

Cahill, Sean, S. Wade Taylor, Steven A. Elsesser, Leandro Mena, DeMarc Hickson, and Kenneth H. Mayer. 2017. "Stigma, Medical Mistrust, and Perceived Racism May Affect PrEP Awareness and Uptake in Black Compared to White Gay and Bisexual Men in Jackson, Mississippi and Boston, Massachusetts." *AIDS Care* 29, no. 11 (November): 1351–58. https://doi.org/10.1080/09540121.2017.1300633.

Cairns, Gus P., Kane Race, and Pedro Goicochea. 2016. "PrEP: Controversy, Agency and Ownership." *Journal of the International AIDS Society* 19, no. 7S6: 21120. https://doi.org/10.7448/IAS.19.7.21120.

Calabrese, Sarah K. 2020. "Understanding, Contextualizing, and Addressing PrEP Stigma to Enhance PrEP Implementation." *Current HIV/AIDS Reports* 17, no. 6 (December): 579–88. https://doi.org/10.1007/s11904-020-00533-y.

Calabrese, Sarah K., Valerie A. Earnshaw, Douglas S. Krakower, Kristen Underhill, Wilson Vincent, Manya Magnus, Nathan B. Hansen, et al.2018. "A Closer Look at Racism and Heterosexism in Medical Students' Clinical Decision-Making Related to HIV Pre-Exposure Prophylaxis (PrEP): Implications for PrEP Education." *AIDS & Behavior* 22, no. 4 (April): 1122–38. https://doi.org/10.1007/s10461-017-1979-z.

Calabrese, Sarah K., and Kristen Underhill. 2015. "How Stigma Surrounding the Use of HIV Preexposure Prophylaxis Undermines Prevention and Pleasure: A Call to Destigmatize 'Truvada Whores.'" *American Journal of Public Health* 105, no. 10 (October): 1960–64. https://doi.org/10.2105/AJPH.2015.302816.

Campbell, Danielle M., Cheriko A. Boone, Michael Chancley, Raniyah Copeland, Kenyon Farrow, Abraham Johnson, Leisha McKinley-Beach, John Meade, Jr, Stacy W. Smallwood, and Justin Smith. "For Us by Us: PrEP in Black America." Black Public Health Academy, February 7, 2023. https://www.treatmentactiongroup.org/publication/for-us-by-us-prep-in-black-america.

Campbell, Jessica T., Olivia R. Adams, Margaret Bennett-Brown, Brennan Woodward, Amanda N. Gesselman, and Gregory Carter. "PrEP Familiarity, Interest, and Usage Among 364 Black and Hispanic Adults in Indiana." *Frontiers in Public Health* 10 (May 6, 2022): 810042. https://doi.org/10.3389/fpubh.2022.810042.

Centers for Disease Control and Prevention. 2023. "HIV and African American Gay and Bisexual Men." Centers for Disease Control and Prevention, February. https://www.cdc.gov/hiv/group/msm/bmsm.html.

———. 2023, May 23. *Diagnoses of HIV Infection in the United States and Dependent Areas, 2021*. Centers for Disease Control and Prevention. https://www.cdc.gov/hiv/library/reports/hiv-surveillance/vol-34/index.html

Commissioner, Office of the. 2021. "FDA Approves First Injectable Treatment for HIV Pre-Exposure Prevention." FDA. FDA, December. https://www.fda.gov/news-events/press-announcements/fda-approves-first-injectable-treatment-hiv-pre-exposure-prevention.

Dehlin, Jessica M., Ryan Stillwagon, Jim Pickett, Lance Keene, and John A. Schneider. 2019. "#PrEP4Love: An Evaluation of a Sex-Positive HIV Prevention Campaign."

JMIR Public Health and Surveillance 5, no. 2 (June): e12822. https://doi.org/10.2196/12822.

Dubov, Alex, Phillip Galbo, Frederick L. Altice, and Liana Fraenkel.2018. "Stigma and Shame Experiences by MSM Who Take PrEP for HIV Prevention: A Qualitative Study." *American Journal of Men's Health* 12, no. 6 (November): 1843–54. https://doi.org/10.1177/1557988318797437.

Earnshaw, Valerie A., and Stephenie R. Chaudoir. 2009. "From Conceptualizing to Measuring HIV Stigma: A Review of HIV Stigma Mechanism Measures." *AIDS and Behavior* 13, no. 6 (December): 1160. https://doi.org/10.1007/s10461-009-9593-3.

Eaton, Lisa A., Seth C. Kalichman, Devon Price, Stephanie Finneran, Aerielle Allen, and Jessica Maksut. 2017. "Stigma and Conspiracy Beliefs Related to Pre-Exposure Prophylaxis (PrEP) and Interest in Using PrEP Among Black and White Men and Transgender Women Who Have Sex with Men." *AIDS and Behavior* 21, no. 5 (May): 1236–46. https://doi.org/10.1007/s10461-017-1690-0.

Edelman, E. Jennifer, Brent A. Moore, Sarah K. Calabrese, Gail Berkenblit, Chinazo Cunningham, Viraj Patel, Karran Phillips, et al. 2017. "Primary Care Physicians' Willingness to Prescribe HIV Pre-Exposure Prophylaxis for People Who Inject Drugs." *AIDS and Behavior* 21, no. 4 (April): 1025–33. https://doi.org/10.1007/s10461-016-1612-6.

Fauci, Anthony S., and H. Clifford Lane. 2020. "Four Decades of HIV/AIDS—Much Accomplished, Much to Do." *New England Journal of Medicine* 383, no. 1 (July): 1–4. https://doi.org/10.1056/NEJMp1916753.

Fauci, Anthony S., Robert R. Redfield, George Sigounas, Michael D. Weahkee, and Brett P. Giroir. 2019. "Ending the HIV Epidemic: A Plan for the United States." *JAMA* 321, no. 9 (March):

Golden, Shelley D., Kenneth R. McLeroy, Lawrence W. Green, Jo Anne L. Earp, and Lisa D. Lieberman. 2015. "Upending the Social Ecological Model to Guide Health Promotion Efforts Toward Policy and Environmental Change." *Health Education & Behavior* 42, no. 1_suppl (April): 8S-14S. https://doi.org/10.1177/1090198115575098.

Golub, Sarit A. 2018. "PrEP Stigma: Implicit and Explicit Drivers of Disparity." *Current HIV/AIDS Reports* 15, no. 2 (April): 190–97. https://doi.org/10.1007/s11904-018-0385-0.

Grant, Robert M, and Kimberly A Koester. 2016. "What People Want From Sex and PrEP." *Current Opinion in HIV and AIDS* 11, no. 1 (January): 3–9. https://doi.org/10.1097/COH.0000000000000216.

Hartmann, Miriam, Michele Lanham, Thesla Palanee-Phillips, Florence Mathebula, Elizabeth E. Tolley, Dean Peacock, Laura Pascoe, et al. 2019. "Generating Charisma: Development Of An Intervention To HelpAnd SafetyIn Their HIV Prevention." *AIDS Education and Prevention: Official Publication of the International Society for AIDS Education* 31, no. 5 (October): 433–51. https://doi.org/10.1521/aeap.2019.31.5.433.

Huang, Ya-lin A., Weiming Zhu, Dawn K. Smith, Norma Harris, and Karen W. Hoover. 2018. "HIV Pre Exposure Prophylaxis, by Race and Ethnicity—United

States, 2014–2016." *MMWR. Morbidity and Mortality Weekly Report* 67, no. 41 (October): 1147–50. https://doi.org/10.15585/mmwr.mm6741a3.

Irungu, Elizabeth, Nomhle Khoza, and Jennifer Velloza. 2021. "Multi-Level Interventions to Promote Oral Pre-Exposure Prophylaxis Use Among Adolescent Girls and Young Women: A Review of Recent Research." *Current HIV/AIDS Reports* 18, no. 6 (December): 490–99. https://doi.org/10.1007/s11904-021-00576-9.

Kamitani, Emiko, Yuko Mizuno, Julia B. DeLuca, and Charles B. Jr Collins. 2023. "Systematic Review of Alternative HIV Preexposure Prophylaxis Care Delivery Models to Improve Preexposure Prophylaxis Services." *AIDS* 37, no. 10 (August): 1593. https://doi.org/10.1097/QAD.0000000000003601.

Keen, Phillip, and Benjamin R. Bavinton. 2020. "Could Disparities in PrEP Uptake Limit the Public Health Benefit?" *The Lancet Public Health* 5, no. 9 (September): e467–68. https://doi.org/10.1016/S2468-2667(20)30183–3.

Keene, Lance C., Jessica M. Dehlin, Jim Pickett, Kathryn R. Berringer, Iman Little, Ashley Tsang, Alida M. Bouris, and John A. Schneider. 2021. "#PrEP4Love: Success and Stigma Following Release of the First Sex-Positive PrEP Public Health Campaign." *Culture, Health & Sexuality* 23, no. 3 (March): 397–413. https://doi.org/10.1080/13691058.2020.1715482.

Louisiana Health Hub—STD/HIV/Hepatitis Program. *TelePrEP*. (2023, August 30). https://www.louisianahealthhub.org/teleprep/.

Marks, Sarah J., Roland C. Merchant, Melissa A. Clark, Tao Liu, Joshua G. Rosenberger, Jose Bauermeister, and Kenneth H. Mayer. 2017. "Potential Healthcare Insurance and Provider Barriers to Pre-Exposure Prophylaxis Utilization Among Young Men Who Have Sex with Men." *AIDS Patient Care and STDs* 31, no. 11 (November): 470–78. https://doi.org/10.1089/apc.2017.0171.

Mayer, Kenneth H., Allison Agwu, and David Malebranche. 2020. "Barriers to the Wider Use of Pre-Exposure Prophylaxis in the United States: A Narrative Review." *Advances in Therapy* 37, no. 5 (May): 1778–1811. https://doi.org/10.1007/s12325-020-01295-0.

McLeroy, Kenneth R., Daniel Bibeau, Allan Steckler, and Karen Glanz. 1988. "An Ecological Perspective on Health Promotion Programs." *Health Education Quarterly* 15, no. 4 (December): 351–77. https://doi.org/10.1177/109019818801500401.

McMahan, Vanessa M., Aleks Martin, Lindsay Garske, Lauren R. Violette, Michele P. Andrasik, Jared M. Baeten, Caleb Banta-Green, and Joanne D. Stekler. 2019. "Development of a Targeted Educational Intervention to Increase Pre-Exposure Prophylaxis Uptake among Cisgender Men and Transgender Individuals Who Have Sex with Men and Use Methamphetamine in Seattle (WA, USA)." *Sexual Health*. https://doi.org/10.1071/SH18060.

McNulty, Moira C., M. Ellen Acree, Jared Kerman, H. Herukhuti Sharif Williams, and John A. Schneider. 2022. "Shared Decision Making for HIV Pre-Exposure Prophylaxis (PrEP) with Black Transgender Women." *Culture, Health & Sexuality* 24, no. 8 (August): 1033–46. https://doi.org/10.1080/13691058.2021.1909142.

Ming, Kristin, Isha Shrestha, Alexander Vazquez, James Wendelborn, Veronica Jimenez, Nadra Lisha, Torsten B. Neilands, et al. 2020. "Improving the HIV PrEP

Continuum of Care Using an Intervention for Healthcare Providers: A Stepped-Wedge Study Protocol." *BMJ Open* 10, no. 7 (July): e040734. https://doi.org/10.1136/bmjopen-2020–040734.

National Institutes of Health. (2021). *Pre-exposure prophylaxis (PrEP)*. https://hivinfo.nih.gov/understanding-hiv/fact-sheets/pre-exposure-prophylaxis-prep.

"New PrEP Formulation Approved . . . but Only for Some." 2019. *The Lancet HIV* 6, no. 11 (November): e723. https://doi.org/10.1016/S2352-3018(19)30350–9.

Nicol, Melanie R., Jessica L. Adams, and Angela Dm Kashuba. 2013. "HIV Pre-Exposure Prophylaxis Trials: The Road to Success." *Clinical Investigation* 3, no. 3 (March): 295–308. https://doi.org/10.4155/cli.12.155.

Pinto, Rogério M., Kathryn R. Berringer, Rita Melendez, and Okeoma Mmeje. 2018. "Improving PrEP Implementation Through Multilevel Interventions: A Synthesis of the Literature." *AIDS and Behavior* 22, no. 11 (November): 3681–91. https://doi.org/10.1007/s10461-018-2184-4.

Quinn, Katherine, Lisa Bowleg, and Julia Dickson-Gomez. 2019. "The Fear of Being Black plus the Fear of Being Gay': The Effects of Intersectional Stigma on PrEP Use among Young Black Gay, Bisexual, and Other Men Who Have Sex with Men." *Social Science & Medicine* 232 (July): 86–93. https://doi.org/10.1016/j.socscimed.2019.04.042.

Sewell, Whitney C., Patricia Solleveld, Dominika Seidman, Christine Dehlendorf, Julia L. Marcus, and Douglas S. Krakower. 2021. "Patient-Led Decision-Making for HIV Preexposure Prophylaxis." *Current HIV/AIDS Reports* 18, no. 1 (February): 48–56. https://doi.org/10.1007/s11904-020-00535-w.

Shrestha, Roman, and Michael Copenhaver. 2018. "Exploring the Use of Pre-Exposure Prophylaxis (PrEP) for HIV Prevention Among High-Risk People Who Use Drugs in Treatment." *Frontiers in Public Health* 6 (July): 195. https://doi.org/10.3389/fpubh.2018.00195.

Siegler, Aaron J., Farah Mouhanna, Robertino Mera Giler, Kevin Weiss, Elizabeth Pembleton, Jodie Guest, Jeb Jones, et al. 2018. "The Prevalence of Pre-Exposure Prophylaxis Use and the Pre-Exposure Prophylaxis–to-Need Ratio in the Fourth Quarter of 2017, United States." *Annals of Epidemiology* 28, no. 12 (December): 841–49. https://doi.org/10.1016/j.annepidem.2018.06.005.

Spieldenner, A. 2016. "Prep whores and HIV prevention: The Queer Communication of HIV Pre-Exposure Prophylaxis (prep)." *Journal of Homosexuality* 63, no. 12 1685–1697. https://doi.org/10.1080/00918369.2016.1158012.

Storholm, Erik D., Allison J. Ober, Matthew L. Mizel, Luke Matthews, Matthew Sargent, Ivy Todd, Deborah Zajdman, and Hank Green. 2021. "Primary Care Providers' Knowledge, Attitudes, and Beliefs About HIV Pre-Exposure Prophylaxis (PrEP): Informing Network-Based Interventions." *AIDS Education and Prevention* 33, no. 4 (August): 325–44. https://doi.org/10.1521/aeap.2021.33.4.325.

Sullivan, Patrick S., Robertino Mera Giler, Farah Mouhanna, Elizabeth S. Pembleton, Jodie L. Guest, Jeb Jones, Amanda D. Castel, et al. 2018. "Trends in the Use of Oral Emtricitabine/Tenofovir Disoproxil Fumarate for Pre-Exposure Prophylaxis against HIV Infection, United States, 2012–2017." *Annals of Epidemiology* 28, no. 12 (December): 833–40. https://doi.org/10.1016/j.annepidem.2018.06.009.

Sullivan, Patrick S., Leandro Mena, Latesha Elopre, and Aaron J. Siegler. 2019. "Implementation Strategies to Increase PrEP Uptake in the South." *Current HIV/AIDS Reports* 16, no. 4 (August): 259–69. https://doi.org/10.1007/s11904-019-00447-4.

Turner, Leah, Abbey Roepke, Emily Wardell, and Anne M. Teitelman. 2018. "Do You PrEP? A Review of Primary Care Provider Knowledge of PrEP and Attitudes on Prescribing PrEP." *Journal of the Association of Nurses in AIDS Care*, HIV Prevention, 29, no. 1 (January): 83–92. https://doi.org/10.1016/j.jana.2017.11.002.

UNAIDS Fact Sheet Global HIV & AIDS Statistics. https://www.unaids.org/en/resources/fact-sheet. Accessed September 14, 2023.

Chapter 5

"You Don't Get Injured on a Shrimp Boat"

Masculinity, Injury, and Agency among Commercial Fishers in the Lowcountry

Jennifer Sweeney Tookes, Tracy Yandle, and Bryan Fluech

In a rural coastal Georgia county, one of the local shrimpers is also the fire chief. When fishers are injured, they tend to call him rather than 911. Sometimes this turns out to be the best move, as a shrimper in his late seventies discovered in 2020. The fire chief related this story:

> I got a phone call from [a shrimper], and . . . in a very faint voice, but kind of high pitched "Help me, I'm dying" and the phone hung up. I looked at my phone. I said "Do you know where he must be? Evidently he's at the dock." I tried to call him back, didn't get no answer. So I jumped into the truck and I run down there. He was laying on the next boat over [from his boat] and there was a trail of blood coming from his boat all the way over. He lay on his back and he was gasping for air, holding his chest, and had his hand behind his back. He had rolled over sideways and he was . . . just trying to breathe. I hear a sucking sound.
>
> He said, "I fell off the roof backwards and landed on the pin rail." So that's when I looked around and pulled him up, and I took a sandwich bag [that he found lying on the boat nearby] and stuck it on the on the second channel of the hole, to keep the lung from collapsing. And it was filled with blood, blood to start to come out of the hole.

> I called 911 and told them that he had fell and impaled himself. I jumped up, [and] got another boy . . . to hold him like that while I went to look for the "mechanism of injury" to see what had hurt him. When I went to the pin rail I found there was meat, a chunk of meat sticking out of the top of the pin rail with blood all over it. I looked down in it and grabbed it and pulled it out and it came out as a core. I looked up above and there was a bloody . . . handprint on the pipe right up above him . . . about three foot above his head where he was laying backwards over it. He fell off the roof backwards, impaled him and it went through. He pulled himself off of that five-six inch [long] pipe that he was impaled on his back! . . . I got all that and I went over there and I said, "Did you pull yourself off of it?" 'He said "yes," and I just said "my goodness!"
>
> So I called to dispatch because they needed to get a life flight helicopter right away because it was a traumatic injury . . . so I had them land right there in the middle of [the park], and they flew him out to Jacksonville.

He later added to this story, describing this "core" that he removed from the pipe where he could "see skin, and then muscle, and then a piece of, like a bone—and I figured that was the shoulder blade under there where it went through. And then there was some more tissue and cartilage, and then another bone—looked like maybe a rib or something." He reported that when the shrimper arrived in the trauma center in Jacksonville that he was close to bleeding out, and the medical team had said he would have died in about "five minutes." This shrimper was walking the halls of the hospital in less than two days, and home within a week. Before a month was over, he was back on his vessel and out shrimping. When asked about this event later, his response was flippant "I shoved a piece of pipe, one inch pipe in my back. Went along, took out seven ribs and almost bit the dust, but we survived it. So, we still kickin'."

His response exemplifies attitudes that have arisen in the context of injuries that occur among commercial fishermen of the Georgia and South Carolina coasts, an area that comprises the central portion of the Lowcountry. This chapter addresses commercial fishers in this region and their perspectives and behaviors around injuries and healthcare-seeking behaviors. It is based in long-term, ethnographic fieldwork with the same community over a span of over ten years. Despite health only being a minor focus for a few small periods of time in this decade, data on the topic has emerged usually unexpectedly, and often unsolicited as part of numerous overlapping and sometimes simultaneous projects. Based on the principles of grounded theory (Glaser and Strauss 1967) these unsolicited explanations were later examined and analyzed through the lenses of medical anthropology, public health, and theories about the body as object, gender performativity, and agency, as articulated below.

LITERATURE

Social Determinants or Assemblages of Health

The World Health Organization explains that conditions into which people are born, grow to adulthood, live, and work influence their health and longevity throughout their lives. These are referred to as social determinants of health (WHO 2023). Factors like socioeconomic status, education, neighborhood and physical environment, employment, and social support networks, as well as access to healthcare, determine lifelong health, and influence how individuals interact with system of care, or are excluded from effective healthcare (WHO 2023).

Recent critiques in medical anthropology have shifted analyses from the rigidity of separate and linear categories used in applications of social determinants of health into an "assemblage model," acknowledging ever-shifting multiplicity and indeterminacy of the lived experience, which more accurately represents human lives and circumstances (Chenhall and Senior 2017; Parsons 2022). An assemblage approach allows us to consider the multilayered connections and interactions between the environmental, political, economic, and social processes in individuals' lives (Chenhall and Senior 2017).

Health of Fishers

Commercial fishing is one of the most dangerous occupations in the United States. Data from the Centers for Disease Control and the National Institute for Occupational Safety and Health show that between 2000 and 2015, the average US worker death rate was four deaths per every 100,000 US workers (CDC 2023). However, in the United States, the fisher death rate during this same period was 117 per 100,000 workers (CDC 2023). This increased rate relates to the challenging work conditions of the industry, with the top causes of injuries and fatalities being work-related accidents, cardiovascular disease, and cancer that are associated with hazardous working conditions, strenuous labor, long work hours, and the impacts of harsh weather conditions.

Fishers are cognizant of the health risks inherent to their profession, and in fact, those with higher income levels elect to purchase health insurance (Crosson 2016). However, they are often unable to purchase health insurance because of the insurance industry's perception of risk and their unwillingness to provide coverage (Light 1992).

Concern about job-related injuries and stressors for fishers has been the focus of considerable study (Lincoln et al. 2021; Kucera et al. 2021; Janocha 2012), and the literature demonstrates that fishers do not generally experience excellent health. In addition to injuries and musculoskeletal strain, fishermen have high mortality from cardiovascular disease and cancer which are largely due to smoking, overweight, and high cholesterol (Pougnet et al. 2013).

Health and safety programs for fisher health in the United States generally focus on injuries that occur during the course of fishing (OSHA 2011; GAO 2022). Elsewhere, Soleo et al. (2013) have focused on efforts in Italy to improve health surveillance in commercial fishing. In Norway, government licensing of fishers has begun to include elements relating to their health and well-being, purportedly to decrease risk of death in the profession. Sonvinsen et al. argue that it has effectively removed hundreds of commercial fishers from legally fishing because of nutrition-related chronic disease and metabolic syndrome. They liken this governmental oversight to Foucault's theory of the "body politic" with the state exercising control over bodies (Sonvinsen et al. 2017)

Agency and the Body

Theorist Michel Foucault's concept of the "body politic" (1977) emphasizes that broad cultural and political power in a society often operates through the regulation and discipline of bodies. These circumscriptions shape behavior and limit individual choices, or *agency*. Anthropologists use *agency* to refer to the capacity of an individual to act and exert choices within specific social and cultural contexts. A focus on individual agency within larger societal or cultural structures illustrates that people do not simply passively react to social forces, but instead actively shape their own lives and negotiate their roles within broader systems of meaning and power.

Similarly, Clifford Geertz (1973) argues that agency emerges in the interchange between cultural *meaning* and individual action, particularly in how individuals interpret and assign significance to social norms and values. Likewise, Pierre Bourdieu's articulation of habitus emphasizes the ways individuals are shaped by their cultural backgrounds and life experiences, and their integration of cultural norms and structures into this worldview (1977). In examining habitus, we can view individuals both reproducing and challenging social structures, while utilizing their own agency to negotiate their positions and actions within a larger environment.

Ethnographic illustrations of agency paired with insights from Geertz, Bourdieu, and Foucault can provide insight into how individuals navigate, or resist, cultural, social, and political expectations. This interplay can illuminate complex dynamics of individual agency in societal contexts and highlight the potential for resistance within structures of power and control. Nancy Scheper-Hughes and Locke explore this idea using the concept of the "social body" as one that has been properly trained, explaining that "Cultures are disciplines that provide codes and social scripts for the domestication of the individual body in conformity to the needs of the social and political order" (1987, 26). Individual agency allows that body to negotiate those codes and scripts while functioning within the social and political order.

Gender Performativity and Pain

This constant negotiation between individual agency and broader societal expectations is exemplified in ethnographic work with undocumented male laborers in San Francisco (Walter, Bourgois, and Loinaz 2004). The authors argue that masculinity itself is a cultural product that is continually reshaped by relationships between individuals as well as by changing macro-power inequalities, thus articulating (without explicitly naming) a sort of "masculine agency." Gender identity is not a static condition, but rather one that is performed and reinforced through interactions with others (Butler 1990; Walter, Bourgois, and Loinaz 2004).

As Judith Butler has articulated, and others have expanded, there is cultural imperative to enact gender, or in this case, manliness. This happens repeatedly through a succession of single events, to build a gender identity via what Butler identifies as a "series of acts which are renewed, revised, and consolidated through time" (1990, 274). In the case of the migrant laborers in San Francisco, masculinity is constructed through the patriarchal accomplishment of financially providing for wives and children back in their home/sending country, and reinforced through their ability to engage in hard physical labor. In their daily quest for paid labor they consciously adjust their stances to "project the image of having a strong, healthy body eager for hard, honest labor" (Walter, Bourgois, and Loinaz 2004, 1161). These men experience conflict between their ability to perform masculinity through labor and financial provision when they are injured and unable to work. In these situations, the "injured workers suddenly fail both as providers and as engaged fathers [as] . . . their worthwhile masculine identity collapses [as] . . . any suggestion of physical impairment dooms one's chances for employment" (Walter, Bourgois, and Loinaz 2004, 1164). If unable to perform masculinity in these culturally accepted manners, their self-perception of male-ness is threatened.

Debra Martin finds similar performativity in the defining of masculinity in relation to violence arguing that "neither violence nor masculinity is fixed and static, but, rather, both are essentially the result of complex behaviors that are relational and dynamic and have power and meaning that is context dependent" (2021, S171). Martin connects this enactment of maleness to an ability to withstand pain, demonstrated via stick fighting carried out by males of the Suri people of Ethiopia. Masculinity and virility were demonstrated by scars and ability to resist acknowledging pain during these violent events (Martin 2021, S173).

Resistance of pain emerges as a key point of occupational culture for professional ballet dancers. They engage with physical pain and suffering as a component of their chosen profession, learn to accept that pain, and in some ways, even embrace it as evidence of their dedication and eligibility for belonging in the field. Anna Aalten argues that dancers treat their bodies as objects that are controlled by their minds, and thus they can selectively choose which elements of the physical experience they elect to acknowledge. Often, they disregard physical pain, as they are "socialized to accept the body's suffering as an inevitable part of their profession" (Aalten 2007, 117). In this way, pain is accepted as an integral part of this process, and is considered "necessary and even somewhat heroic" (Aalten 2007, 122).

This cognitive process around pain exemplifies the notion of the "mindful body" (Scheper-Hughes and Locke 2007) which posits that pain is acknowledged and expressed in the process of interaction between an individual's feelings and thoughts, and the structural systems of belief in the broader culture around them. The imperative of this strategy for handling pain and injury similarly demonstrates notions of "occupational culture" which explicates the ways that people who share a profession often also subscribe to a similar belief system and behavioral code, including unwritten rules to obey or reactions to express in a given situation (Hochschild, 1983; Clark, Chandler & Barry 1994).

Masculinity and Health

In examining the point of intersection of these broad fields of thought, we find literature on masculinity and health (Evans et al. 2011; Creighton and Oliffe 2010; Broom 2009). Courtenay (2009) argues that social practices—such as health-related beliefs and behaviors—define a space in which masculinity can be demonstrated and performed. Masculinity has been linked to negative health outcomes because of factors such as lower levels of social support and more cardiovascular stressors (Robertson 2007), and men are less likely to make visits to healthcare providers and more likelyto have had no recent contact with physicians (Courtenay 2009). The literature demonstrates that men are also more likely to enact and negotiate masculinity via hard physical labor, the ability to ignore pain, and to reject healthcare in pursuit of a more masculine social image (Courtenay 2009). These theoretical perspectives coalesce in field research among commercial fishers of the southeastern United States.

Local Context

The US states of Georgia and South Carolina hug either side of the Savannah River basin, and many of the coastal counties in these two Atlantic states are classified as "rural." People living in rural areas of the United States experience poorer health outcomes than their urban counterparts. Health disparities in these rural areas are linked to lack of access to healthcare services, healthcare provider shortages, lower rates of health insurance, and lower educational and socioeconomic and statuses (Bergeron et al. 2013). According to the U.S. Census Bureau, between 10 and 30 percent of the people in these counties are living below the poverty threshold (2021).

Commercial fishing has been a significant economic and cultural component of the history and heritage of this region. The extensive network of salt marshes and prolific estuaries, beaches, and coastal zones in this region have supported shrimping and trapping of blue crabs for generations. Fishers have also targeted fish such as snapper, grouper, and seabass, as well as harvested clams and oysters along the shores. Cannonball jellyfish for export to Asian markets are the newest addition to the landings, and have been a financial support for shrimpers when the shrimp season is closed. Many of these businesses were established generations ago, with sons and daughters fishing, shrimping, or selling seafood with their parents and grandparents.

Historically many of the fishing communities in the Lowcountry were Gullah Geechee communities, people who are considered (not undisputedly) to be the descendants of the enslaved Africans who were forced to work the rice, indigo, and cotton plantations of marshes, estuaries, and barrier islands between the Cape Fear River in North Carolina and the St. John's River near Jacksonville, Florida, an area collectively called the "Lowcountry" (Matory 2008). It is important to note these communities have been economically marginalized from fishing since the 1930s, but many are still actively harvesting seafood today.

Today US seafood production operates under strict regulation and management. The ocean waters closest to shore (generally 0–3 miles) are regulated by state agencies, while the span from 3–200 miles typically falls under federal fisheries management, based on the Magnuson-Stevens Fishery Conservation and Management Act. Fisheries management in the United States is mandated to set maximum catch levels based on science and has successfully rebuilt 40 stocks since 2007. However, while progress has been made in ecosystem restoration, the economic viability of fisheries remains a concern. Regulatory structures since the 1990s have imposed restrictions on US fishers, limiting the volume and variety of fish species they can catch. At the same time, fuel costs have increased, and international competition has led to lower fish prices (Tookes, Yandle, and Barlett 2018). As a result, the commercial fishing industry has declined, discouraging new entrants. Currently, the vast majority of the activity fishing and shrimping fleet in this region is male and prefers the term "fishermen" (although one women did explain that she feels her identity as a "shrimper" circumvents this question) (Branch and Kleiber 2015).

METHODS

The authors have conducted mixed method, longitudinal research in the commercial fishing communities of the southeastern Atlantic states of Georgia and South Carolina since 2013. A variety of intersecting and adjacent research projects have allowed the researchers to conduct over a hundred structured, semi-structured, and unstructured interviews in these areas, as well as countless hours of participant observation. Only one project focused specifically on health and well-being among southeastern fishing crew (Yandle, Tookes, and Shamshak 2019), and participants in that study were asked "are there common injuries that occur in commercial fishing?" and "What do fishers or their crew do if they are injured while on a boat?"

While illness and injuries have not been the focus of the vast majority of the interviews conducted in the region, participants have repeatedly volunteered information relevant to this topic. The long-term, intensive ethnographic research in the community began to reveal intriguing commonalities in the ways that injury and illness were described and portrayed by commercial fishers. Once this focus presented itself, the researchers returned to their database of 101 interview transcripts to code specifically for topics relating to injury and illness. The data discussed in this chapter is the result of this secondary analysis.

FINDINGS

Work Ethic and Reliability

Strong work ethic is a cultural value that arises very commonly—fishers acknowledge that fishing is extremely physically (and sometimes psychologically) demanding work, and maintain that being able to work hard for long hours is not only vital, but common. Reliable and hardworking captains and crew are respected and do not have trouble staying employed. Similarly, fishers and crew who are not willing to engage in strenuous physical labor in the humid, hot southern sun do not last in the industry. Word of this "laziness" travels rapidly through the community. Many fishers we interviewed explained the importance of a strong work ethic to contextualize their enculturation to fishing boat culture, particularly around topics of illness and injury.

Seasickness

When fishers recount their early days in fishing, many begin with stories of experiencing nausea induced by being on the water. Sometimes this seasickness was difficult at first, but then the fisher would acclimate to the sea and no longer be bothered by it. "My cousin, he was on the shrimp boat, and my brother growing up. I wanted to see what it was like and when I went out with him, I got seasick, and I lay on the floor. They'd bring me back after they get through and I'd go right back and fight it out, kind of got used to it, it worked out pretty good." Another fisher took a bit longer in his adjustment period: "I remember getting sick growing up, all through kindergarten to age ten, and then, finally, it was like at age ten, a switch flipped with me because, 'hey, you got to work, you don't have time to get sick!'" He explained that when he was hanging over the side of the boat "the crew would actually hold me by my belt to be sure I wouldn't fall over if something was to happen because you might hit a log and it jar the boat, the wind might gust and the boat roll or something." Each of these men eventually overcame nausea and became productive members of the crew.

In a few cases, the stories of the seasickness experience were dramatic:

> I can't remember how old I was, there was a day I told my dad, "I'm going shrimping with you," and he said, "No son, you don't need to. There's going to be a nor'easter . . . seas are going to be kind of rough. You don't need to go. You'll get sick." And I did, but I went anyway. And my grandfather called over to the radio on him and said, "You need to carry that boy home. He's sick." And Daddy said, "No, I ain't doing it. This is the most shrimp I've caught all week. I told him not to come. He's going to learn." Well I did, I guess . . . I didn't die.

The misery of seasickness came through clearly in one fisherman's story, as he told the researchers:

> You can't explain seasickness. I can't explain it but I tell you what, if you ever been seasick you know what I'm talkin' about. I've been seasick a month straight. Every day, when I eat in the morning I had to try to lay down quick before I threw up . . . that first night when we got offshore, oh my gosh, I got sick and I stayed sick for probably over a month. Every day, every night, throwing up, throwing up, throwing up, every night. I couldn't come home, 'cause it took us three days and three nights to get there, and Daddy wasn't going to bring me back home. So, you was there, when you got out there, you was *there*. And

> you stick it out until you finally get over it, and I got over it. The rougher it got, the better I felt then, after that.

Another described a different fisherman he had worked with, who had "been out at sea and he was seasick so long, the captain came to him and he said he was so sick he felt like he was going to die! Captain told him, says, 'I've never known anybody die from seasickness.' 'Oh Lord, Captain, I thought I was gonna die. I thought dying would be a relief to me!'"

In each of these stories, the unwavering dedication to completing the task rather than giving up and returning to shore—even in the face of miserable and debilitating nausea—reinforces this notion of work ethic being valued above all personal distress. As independent fishermen, none of whom answered to a supervisor or "boss," each of them could feasibly have chosen to return their ill colleagues or children to shore. Yet, in each case, this was not considered to be an acceptable solution, as it would require admitting that personal well-being was important, and that the individual did not have the fortitude to overcome the misery. This lack of concern was summarized by one captain, who emphatically informed the author "So far as being sick like just like pukin' or somethin' like that? You got to deal with it till we go home. *Yes, ma'am*!"

"Minor" Injuries

Fishers get sick and injured on the job. Beyond simple seasickness, their fingers, hands, and limbs get smashed or dismembered. They suffer broken bones from slipping, falling, or objects smashing into them. At times, they fall from the roof of the wheelhouse or the rigging, and not always into the more forgiving surface of the water. When asked about typical injuries, the most common responses centered around minor cuts, bites, and stabs, such as these:

- "I've been bitten shark bit. Stingrays put two or three hooks in my fingers."
- "Just creaks and cuts, [like] shrimp horns, stingray pokes, getting bitten or cut by a fish, jellyfish sting . . . it's no big deal [but] your hands get wore out and blistered."
- "Common injuries [are] hooks in the hand, or knife cuts . . . you know hands are scarred over and feel like sandpaper all the time . . . we wear gloves but . . . you can't keep them tight right? So you get blisters on your hands."
- "I've heard some of 'em getting bit by a shark or whatever."

- "The only thing I've ever heard of in terms of injuries, for the most part is someone being careless with fish or sharks."
- "Most times not too many people get hurt. You get your cuts, and stuff like that."

Less glamorous, but just as common are the issues resulting from repetitive, hard labor in challenging environmental conditions. A crabber explained his own struggles: "[My] back was getting pretty bad. I was working really hard . . . The doctor did an MRI and said 'Oh, well, I see what the problem is!' He says 'Most people have got 12 lower lumbar vertebra. You got 13!' I said 'Well damn, why am I so short?!' Well they say . . . in between my 12th and 13th lumbar vertebra was probably beaten [apart] in the boat" and all the nerves are compacted in that region of his back. He said he is currently implementing his own version of physical therapy in hopes of avoiding surgery.

Another explained that his "knees bother me a little bit" which he attributes to being "beaten up through the years." He noted that this pressure on his body had even noticeably compacted his joints, making him shorter: "I used to be six-foot-tall and I been up on that boat for forty-five years!" These type of repetitive, long-term injuries are often dismissed by fishers like this one: "We all get them. I mean, I got a knee right now that's messed up. We just pull an anchor one morning when I was probably in my 20s and a block come loose and hit me in the kneecap. Leg prolly swole up big as a basketball . . . [I] didn't go to the doctor but nowadays I feel it. I mean, you get older, you feel old. . . . I broke that finger there prolly six months ago, you see it's all crooked." In each case, these long-term, chronic joint issues are dismissed as being a normal part of aging.

Overboard and Dangers of the Ocean

Injuries and persistent, chronic pain are often downplayed, but a common concern is having people fall off the boat. Sometimes these were fortunately mild events, such as one captain who explained: "I've had a guy fall. [He was] stepping off the boat onto the dock . . . and fell in between, [but it] didn't hurt him. Got him to swim around the back of the boat and got him out in the back of the boat."

A different fisher seems to still be amused by his overboard adventure, as he described falling off the shrimp boat when he was fifteen years old:

> My sister likes to tell about when I got knocked overboard . . . The captain . . . was getting ready to put the rigs out at 5:30 in the morning, it was still dark, . . . and he went and pulled the nets off and pulled the doors off, and then the nets followed them. 99 percent of the time it works fine. But this time it happened

> to catch a cable that swung around and thumped me in the back. It didn't hurt, but it threw me off balance and just flipped me over the rail. So, I was basically swimming in Sapelo Sound and nobody on the boat but my dad and my two sisters. They weren't much help. My dad, instead of calling some of the other boats around saying "Hey! [My son's] in the water can you grab him?" He wasn't gonna do that. He went and got the life ring, and he must have thrown it at least 50 yards. That thing was whistling—it was a hard plastic life ring—and I heard it, and I could see it, and I ducked under the water till I heard it hit the water. If it woulda hit me, it would have killed me! I think he was kind of excited. . . . He would go this way, and he had my sisters say, "Alright, he's over there . . . Now he's over there," and he'd turn the boat around and drive back past me the other way . . . I'd kind of dog-paddle past the boat because I could swim like a fish, it didn't matter to me. It was warm. Then he'd go back that way, then I'd turn around and dog-paddle the other way behind him. It took him about 30 minutes . . . And then he got me a rope, and when I got back on the boat, *then* he told people that I had been in the water. But, he wasn't telling anybody anything till he got me back on that boat! And then we didn't come back to the dock, I think we just went back shrimpin'. We went on to work. No harm, no foul!

Not everyone was as unconcerned about having a person overboard as that father seemed to be. One fisher explained a stressful day at sea with his wife:

> My wife fell over one time, I didn't even know what happened! We'd been fishing, we just dumped our drag, and we was goin' behind the island to take a little break, [to] throw the anchor out and eat lunch. I went back there and she wasn't on the boat. I mean it's the worst feeling I ever had in my life. . . . She was back there tying up a tarp, staying on the back of the boat and the rope she was tying it, she was kind of pulling on it, and it broke. The momentum—she fell in the water. About 10 minutes later, I realized she was gone. I mean, my Lord! I looked back, and I couldn't see her! I panicked, turned round, wide open, headed back to where I come from, and thank the Lord, I seen a little head bobbin' there. . . . Went up there and threw her a life ring and got her back on the boat. That was scary, you wouldn't believe what goes through your mind when something like that happens.

Both of these people who found themselves in the ocean were very fortunate, based on the warnings from a different shrimper, who described the dangers of being on a boat: "You can fall overboard and—sharks! I mean, the sharks follow the boats all the time. You fall in the water, you probably get ate up by a shark. They eat our nets up."

Some of the stories depicted far more frightening situations. One of the older shrimpers in the fleet told us a story about his own terrifying experience prompted by seeing another shrimper he knew:

> [His] daddy saved my life, when I was nineteen years old. I got pulled overboard and pulled unconscious in the shrimp net. Coast Guard said I was dead. [His] daddy kept pumping. They said "you just wasting your time." No offense to you, they say I was just black as a black person. I had no life. He kept pumping. The Coast Guard said "You just wasting your time." He said "I got a whole lotta time." He kept pumping. They done called my family and my wife and told 'em I was dead. They brang me to St. Simon's Pier. But in between that time [thump] he hit the right spot and I come back!

The stories we did not hear in these situations were those that resulted in the death of fishers. Overboard deaths do occur—there were 207 between 2000 and 2016, with over 30 percent of those occurring on the US Atlantic coast—but these fishers were fortunate in their relatively easy rescues (Case, Lincoln, and Lewis 2018), and "tales" that involved fishers who were killed were never volunteered.

Severe and Disfiguring Injuries

Work on commercial fishing vessels can turn from productive to deadly in the blink of an eye. The more unusual injuries are evidently a source of fascination, and are described less flippantly than the minor cuts and stabs. The stories of these injuries are often told like epic tales. One shrimper described his father, saying "We could write a book about him. He's had a compound fracture in this arm and he went fishing four days after —Both his bones come out of his arm and he went shrimping . . . with my four-year-old brother on an 80-foot boat!" The father punctuated that story by whipping off his shoe and showing us that another shrimping adventure resulted in his missing big toe.

Many explained the situation as nonchalantly as this captain: "You got moving parts, you got people, you got accidents! I mean, I've seen them wrapped up in the winch, lose an arm. Luckily no lives. But you know, fingers . . . there've been broken arms and feet and fingers and stuff like that. I mean, that happens." This final statement is often accompanied by a shrug to indicate that it is not considered to be a significant issue, and a comment such as this one: "Just one of those things you have to deal with."

The machinery on the boat is of industrial size and strength, and has the potential to severely harm people: "I know people that have gotten their arms and legs ripped off due to the cables on the winches because they weren't paying attention or messed up." Often the crew members that a fishermen can hire are not long on experience with the vessels. One captain explained a specific day where that lack of experience nearly turned deadly for a man:

> I said, "Now, if you ever get a rope wound up in this spool, *don't fight it*. Stop the winch from turning. That's all you have to do. *Then* you fight it . . . you *stop the thing* that's causing the problem." That's simple as I could put it. [One day] it was causing him a problem. So he steady was fightin' it! I was on the stern of the boat and I couldn't get there quick enough. I hollered, "Turn the winch off, stop the winch!" He panic, he steady fighting. The winch kept turning.

A large block of wood attached to the rope then hit the man and then became wedged in the winch machinery, fortunately right before the crew member was pulled into the winch. He continued "I said 'You could have gotten killed right then!' But he said 'I panicked.' So . . . anybody that got on the boat with me. I would tell them things that could happen. And if it *could* happen, it *would* happen one day. I would tell them things that could hurt. 'Don't do this. Don't do that.' But when you panic . . . Thank God it didn't, cause I think it could've killed him."

An older captain showed us a mark on his forearm where he suffered a deep gash while fishing. He explained that his family made him seek medical treatment because of the depth of the cut, and in fact, the doctors had to reattach the tendons in his arm. Unfortunately, this repair did not stay repaired, as he explained: "Where it was cut in two, they had to go up this way [indicates on his arm] to get the tendons and pull them back down. [At a later date] I was in church for preaching and I was sitting there, my wife and I, and all at once, one [pain] shot up my arm!" This pain was accompanied by a spasm that forced his arm violently and suddenly straight up into the air,

> and if you don't believe I woke everybody up in that church, oh my, bless it. Everybody looked at me because I didn't expect it. I mean I didn't know it was gonna go up there! But I remember that old country song, that squirrel going up a woman's dress. Well, that's what I figured there, one went up my sleeve!. . . . It is terrible to have something like that happen. Unexpected. Just quick. You know, it hurts when it shoots up the arm, it does!

Other times, the cause of infirmity is not as immediately obvious as these dramatic injuries. For example, this shrimper described a crew member with a sudden issue: "We had a guy last January, [the Coast Guard] had to come get him off the boat. He had a seizure. He seized out for six hours. But he never came to the whole time before the Coast Guard got him off the boat. They came and it took them, I don't know, hour and a half or so to even get on the boat." The shrimper wasn't sure of the cause of these seizures, but other fishers have pointed at these types of issues as being related to chemical use.

Prescription Drug Use and Abuse

In many interviews, comments about pain or injuries led to a discussion about drug use. Fishers told us that the abuse of prescription painkillers was common in the industry. One explained:

> back in the day, you know before it became so prevalent and so . . . if they hurt their backs or something . . . then they'd go to the doctor and the doctor would start giving them all these Lorcets. Then [eventually] your body will tell you "Well I'm hurting so you need to keep taking the Lorcet." . . . I don't think any of them ever intended to get hooked on the stuff, some of them did have some injuries and then this little pharmacy in Darian, was 1 out 5 in the nation that was distributing the oxycodone.

This type of scenario, where injury leads to prescription drug use, which leads to continued off-label usage, and subsequent addiction was described by many others as well.

Another vessel-owner agreed with this story, explaining: "I've worked with a lot of captains, there's a lot of good people on the water. There's a lot of people that are . . . on drugs of some sort, alcohol. . . . And I've seen so many people [that could be] better fisherman than I was when I was fishing, but they just couldn't stay away from the drugs and it cost 'em everything. And quite a few of them are dead now. So, it's a sad tale, but I don't know how you fix it." A less verbose fisher summed up the situation by identifying a key problem in the fishing industry: "OxyContin. I just know there's no place for that. There's so many ways that you can get hurt."

Drug use in the industry is common enough that industry insiders discuss the functionality of workers who are under the influence of different types of chemicals. There is a slight bit more empathy for those addicted to prescription opioids, as one man explained: "I've seen pills sneak up on some really good people. Like really good fishermen lose everything they own because they took one pain pill 'cause they had a hurt back and then it just eat 'em up. They gotta have 'em. Versus meth, I mean, I would think that you just gotta *wanna* do drugs if you're going to go smoke the glass pipe, ya know." This distinction in functionality between people using different types of chemicals, or those trying to beat an addiction, is also summarized in this dock manager's description of a new employee on the opioid treatment prescription drug Suboxone:

> This guy that I was working with— he hadn't been working for me for like three weeks. But the first two or three days, I thought he was gonna kill himself, working so hard. I mean he was just like wide open and I knew what it was. He had just gotten on Suboxone, and so he's like, coming off the stuff, and the

> Suboxone really wires you . . . well three weeks later, now he's burn out. And he worked seven days last week. You know . . . we don't normally do that but . . . he says, "I wanna work, I wanna work," and I said, "You can't do this every day. Your body won't let you." [He said] "Oh yeah, I'm alright."He was sick yesterday and now he's totally sick.

Despite the prevalence of opioid use in the industry, no participants have volunteered comments relating to drug treatment centers or programs, just implied that these individual have made their own choices, and are responsible for the consequences of those choices.

Responsibility *for* and Denial *of* Injury

However, concern about safety for others did arise in the context of captain and vessel-owner obligations. We were told repeatedly that it is the captain's responsibility to keep people safe. The captains we have interviewed emphasized that they run a strict vessel to prevent situations that could lead to injury, and that everyone on the boat is looking out for one another in order to prevent harm. One fisher explained: "I mean *I've heard* of people . . . getting hurt on the boat, like a rope pulling the nets and . . . catch their shirt, or sleeve, or something like that. Heard like that on the winch, but other than that, very rarely. Very rarely, but that's the main thing: everybody be trying their best to stay away from injuries. Everybody be looking out for one another."

When asked about common injuries, many of the vessel owners and captains downplayed this potential in order to highlight their own supervisory prevention. One explained: "You got moving parts, you got people. You got accidents. I mean, I've seen them wrapped up in the winch, lose an arm. Luckily no lives. But you know, fingers—like I said *I ain't never had anybody work for me* that left here but I mean, you know there've been broken arms and feet and fingers and stuff like that. I mean, that happens." So while he acknowledges that injuries *do* happen in the industry, he emphasizes that they are not occurring on his boat. Another captain explained this clearly: "On *my boat* anyway, we try to keep it as safe as possible. So nobody does get hurt, you know?"

There are consequences associated with this concern for crew safety. One fisher explained oversight and reporting: "If you're a licensed boat and you have an injury, you have to report that to the Coast Guard." However, this was heard only a single time across the multitude of interviews analyzed from a decade of research. Another boat owner said that "Normally, if we have an injury we try to pay the hospital bill so we don't get sued," so ownership does come with real, financial consequences for unsafe situations. However, one individual contextualized this captain emphasis on safety, explaining a different perspective: "Most of the captains and boat owners . . . if you're up on a riggin' and you fall—*you better be dead when you get to the deck, because if you ain't I'm gonna throw you overboard.* I mean it's just kind of like, a rule of thumb, that *you don't get hurt on a shrimp boat.*" It is the captain's responsibility to keep everyone safe, apparently regardless of the methods of doing this.

What became clear in this analysis, though, is that even when someone *does* get injured, it's not always considered an "injury." Overwhelmingly, our data indicates that medical care is generally avoided. It is considered inconvenient to seek care, and when the topic is discussed, a scornful tone emerges when describing someone who has sought care on their own without clear and obvious need. When asked about an injury that probably should have received medical care, one fisher showed us his hand and explained: "I broke that finger there prolly six months ago. You see its all crooked there? Never went to the doctor or get it fixed, just keep going . . . if ain't something life or death, we'll pretty much ride it out. [It's] just too much aggravation to go in to have something done." Even broken bones aren't always treated by a healthcare provider, although that is something that people may seek care for: "If they get a broken bone they'll *normally* go to the doctor," but even a broken bone doesn't *always* warrant care.

A shrimper recounted a story from his childhood. When he was thirteen years old he went fishing with his father and older brother, got his index finger caught in a rope, and the rope sliced off everything above the tip (distal phalange) of the finger. His father saw this injury (and his younger brother trying to save the finger part in a tub of ice), and wrapped it with a dirty deck rag and duct tape. Then his father told him "That's not a part of your finger you need for shrimping" and continued on with the trip. To this day, the shrimper finds this event amusing rather than traumatic or problematic.

The thought process behind this type of injury and reaction is exemplified in this example of a fisher who deciding how to handle an injury:

> Interviewer: "How bad does an injury have to be or, how bad does the health condition have to be before people actually go and get medical care?"
>
> Fisher: "I mean, just depends on how tough you are . . . I mean, I didn't go to the doc for 'bout a day for when I broke my arm, but like, I just wrapped it up."
>
> Interviewer: "So you were deciding that it wasn't broken?"
>
> Fisher: "Oh, it was broke! I just, I didn't really feel like goin' in at the moment."

An explicit choice was made to prioritize his own "toughness" over his clear understanding of medical necessity.

DISCUSSION

Health Assemblages

Social determinants of health posit that people with lower levels of education and of lower socioeconomic status will have poorer health outcomes. In these communities, the interactions of the features—the assemblage—impacts but does not necessary "predict" outcomes. This study population is comprised of people who are largely lesser-educated. Many of them came of age when fishing was a highly successful, multigenerational family business. At that time, there was little emphasis placed on seeking higher education in these communities. This reality emerges in the demographics of the study population: of more than one hundred fishers this study team has interviewed, only four or five of them have attended any college. The medical resources in rural counties, such as the ones in which many of these fishers live, are poor, leading to decreased health outcomes (Bergeron et al. 2013). Economic stability is a constant concern, as decision-making about financial outlay in medical care has to be balanced with financial investment in their vessels and gear. Vessels and gear have the potential to facilitate great financial gain, but medical care will not. Most fishers we have interviewed do not have medical insurance.

Economic conditions in the commercial fishing industry have been destabilized by changing conditions in fisheries, and the shifts in state and federal regulations that dictate how they can utilize the ocean resources. Many are chafing under their inability to fish the way they (or their fathers and grandfathers) used to, and are impacted by dramatically increasing fuel costs to run their boats, and considerably lower prices for the fish they catch, because of increased market competition from imported seafood (Tookes, Yandle, and Barlett 2018). As a result, incomes for commercial fishers are lower than they were in previous decades.

These factors are not simple predictors of poor health outcomes, but rather, interact with the larger cultural and social constraints on fishers' lives in these communities, to reduce access to (or decrease imperative to seek) healthcare. In this complex set of interactions, we see the multilayered interactions and processes of environmental, political, economic, and social pressures expressed by the assemblage model (Chenhall and Senior 2017; Parsons 2022).

Masculinity and Agency

Regardless of the financial instability, those who remain in the industry are expected to continue to exemplify the work ethic demonstrated by commercial fishers from more financially solvent generations. This is particularly frustrating for those who feel that state and federal management, and regulation of these species and waters, is excessive and overreaches what should be accepted by those who wish to utilize the natural resources of the region. Among fishers there is an undercurrent of rebellion—frequently fishers resist doing things *just because* they are *supposed* to do them, often to their own potential detriment, such as refusing safety advice or checks of their vessels by the Coast Guard. This spirit becomes evident in their frustrated reactions to regulations and management, however, they must comply with these mandates or risk steep fines, losing their permits or vessels, and subsequently, their livelihoods.

Fishers are fiercely independent, and resist efforts to encroach on their autonomy, but their individual freedoms are constrained by forces far beyond their control. Yet, when it comes to their own *physical bodies*, fishers have the opportunity to engage in a battle of wills against *themselves*. Like ballet dancers, who consent to pain and suffering as evidence of dedication to their profession, fishers similarly accept that injuries and chronic pain will be part of their lived experiences as fishers. Refusing to seek medical care is an opportunity to perform a type of masculinity that refuses to acknowledge pain. Each single refusal is one event in the "series of acts which are renewed, revised, and consolidated through time" (Butler 1990). Admitting injury is not manly, and would acknowledge yet another unwanted mandate on their lives.

Every occupation has its own culture (Aalten 2007, 110). People in the same profession usually share a moral belief system and a behavioral code, telling them how to behave and what, usually unwritten, rules to obey (Hochschild, 1983; Clark, Chandler & Barry 1994). Occupational cultural beliefs about injury and illness emerge around questions of agency and responsibility. In commercial fishing, it is ultimately the captain's responsibility to keep people safe. At this troubling intersection, at first there appear to be limited avenues for captains to acknowledge injuries on their vessels: They can either place blame on the person who gets hurt or take responsibility for allowing an unsafe environment. However, the occupational culture of commercial fishing has made space for a third option, and data discussed in this chapter illustrate this alternate path: By emphasizing the criteria for performative masculinity *before* any injuries occur, the industry incentivizes the downplaying of injuries and performative ignoring of physical ailments. This allows space for the slippage between these two categories.

There is a definite atmosphere of distrust and skepticism about people who get injured or ill, and we were told repeatedly that "You don't get injured on a shrimp boat." This leaves choice up to the individual who is injured: Either injury means you were likely careless; and it's your own fault, or you can demonstrate your agency and control over your circumstances, as well as enacting masculinity, by denying the severity of your own injury. So when a father tells his son "that's not a part of your finger you need for shrimping" he is communicating (1) how to be a man in this culture, and (2) bodily concern is not acceptable and does not fit with the needed work ethic in this context.

CONCLUSION

The data in this chapter emerged organically across a multiplicity of adjacent and sometimes interrelated research projects in the central Lowcountry of Georgia and South Carolina over a period of ten years. This type of longitudinal, intensive research with the same communities is the hallmark of the discipline of Anthropology, and reveals truths about the human condition that cannot be discovered, or determined in any other way. There is no efficient route to the types of insights we can elucidate using some of our most traditional methodologies. This paper is an example of the richness of the findings that emerge using this approach.

Analyzing these qualitative interview results for themes relating to injury, gender identity, and healthcare-seeking behaviors revealed multiple links to the existing literature, and can be contextualized with local social systems, assemblage models of health, occupational culture, gender performativity, and masculinity at the intersection of individual agency.

Fishers see their bodies and their control over them, as well as their decision to work through injury, as part of their dedication to the profession, as demonstration of their masculinity, and one last vestige of control over their work in a setting in which that control is increasingly taken from them. As injuries occur, fishers are faced with the choice of how to handle this potentially rich opportunity to display their mastery of occupational culture, their masculinity, and their ability to drown out the physical needs of their body. For many of the fishers in this sample the choice is simple: It "just depends on how tough you are."

REFERENCES CITED

Aalten, Anna. 2007. "Listening to the Dancer's Body." *The Sociological Review* 55, no. 1 (February): 109–25.

Bergeron, Caroline D., Caroline Foster, Daniela B. Friedman, Andrea Tanner, and Sei-Hill Kim. "Clinical Trial Recruitment in Rural South Carolina: A Comparison of Investigators' Perceptions and Potential Participant Eligibility." *Rural and Remote Health* 13, no. 4 (November): 171–84.

Bourdieu, Pierre. 1977. *Outline of a Theory of Practice*. Cambridge: Cambridge University Press.

Branch, Trevor, and Danika Kleiber.2017. "Should We Call Them Fishers or Fishermen?" *Fish and Fisheries* 18 no. 1 (January): 114–27.

Broom, A., and P. Tovey. 2009. "Introduction: Men's Health in Context." In *Men's Health: Body, Identity, & Social Context.* Chichester: Wiley-Blackwell; 1–5.

Butler, Judith. 1990. "Performative Acts and Gender Constitution: An Essay in Phenomenology and Feminist Theory." In *Performing Feminisms: Feminist Critical Theory and Theatre*. Edited by Sue-Ellen Case. Baltimore: Johns Hopkins University Press.

Case, Samantha L, Jennifer M Lincoln, and Devin L Lucas. 2018. "Fatal Falls Overboard in Commercial Fishing—United States, 2000–2016." *MMWR Morbidity and Mortality Weekly Report* 67: 465–69.

Centers for Disease Control. 2023. "Commercial Fishing Safety." National Institute for Occupational Safety and Health. https://www.cdc.gov/niosh/topics/fishing/default.html.

Chenhall, Richard and Kate Senior. 2018. "Living the Social Determinants of Health: Assemblages in a Remote Aboriginal Community." *Medical Anthropology Quarterly* 32 no. 2: 177–95.

Clark, H., J Chandler, and J Barry. 1994. *Organizations and Identities*. London: Chapman and Hall.

Connell, R. W. 1995. *Masculinities*. Berkeley: University of California Press.

Courtenay, Will. 2009. "Theorising Masculinity and Men's Health." In *Men's Health: Body, Identity and Social Context*. edited by Alex Broom and Philip Tovey 9–32, Chichester: Wiley-Blackwell.

Creighton, Genevieve, and John L Oliffe. 2010. "Theorising Masculinities and Men's Health: A Brief History with a View to Practice." *Health Sociology Review* 19, no. 4 (October): 409–18.

Crosson, Scott. 2016. "The Affordable Care Act and Opportunities for Change in North Carolina's Commercial Fisheries." *Marine Resource Economics* 31, no. 2 (January): 121–29.

Evans, Joan, Blye Frank, John L. Oliffe, and David Gregory. 2011. "Health, Illness, Men and Masculinities (HIMM): A Theoretical Framework for Understanding Men and their Health." *Journal of Men's Health* 8, no. 1 (January): 7–15.

Foucault, Michel. 1977. *Discipline and Punish: The Birth of the Prison*. London: Allen Lane.

Georgia Department of Community Affairs. 2021. "Geographic Area Name—Georgia Department of Community Affairs." https://www.dca.ga.gov/sites/default/files/2021_ga_jtc_estimates_final.pdf.

Geertz, Clifford. 1973. *The Interpretation of Cultures: Selected Essays*. New York City: Basic Books.

Glaser, Barney G., and Anselm L. Strauss. 1967. *The Discovery of Grounded Theory; Strategies for Qualitative Research.* Chicago: Aldine Publishing Company.

Gutmann, M. C. 1996. *The Meanings of Macho: Being a Man in Mexico City.* Berkeley: University of California Press.

Hochschild, A.R. 1983. *The Managed Heart.* Berkeley: University of California Press.

Janocha, Jill. 2012. "Facts of the Catch: Occupational Injuries, Illnesses, and Fatalities to Fishing Workers, 2003–2009." *Beyond the Numbers: Workplace Injuries* 1, no. 9 (U.S. Bureau of Labor Statistics, August): https://www.bls.gov/opub/btn/volume-1/facts-of-the-catch-occupational-injuries-illnesses-and-fatalities-to-fishing-workers-2003-2009.htm.

Kucera, Kristen L., Dana Loomis, Hester Lipscomb, and Stephen Marshall. 2010. "Prospective Study of Incident Injuries Among Southeastern United States Commercial Fishermen." *Occupational and Environmental Medicine* 67, no.12 (December):829–36. DOI:10.1136/oem.2009.053140. Epub 2010 Oct 8. PMID: 20935288.

Light, D. W. 1992. "The Practice and Ethics of Risk-rated Health Insurance." *Journal of the American Medical Association* 267, no. 18 (May): 2503–08.

Lincoln, Jennifer M., Ann Carruth, Debra Cherry, Laurel Kincl, and Laura N. Syron. 2021. "Occupational Health Research in the Commercial Fishing Industry." *Journal of Agromedicine*, 26, no. 1 (January):28–30. DOI: 10.1080/1059924X.2021.1849494.

Martin, Debra. 2021. "Violence and Masculinity in Small-Scale Societies." *Current Anthropology* 62, no. S23 (February): 169–81.

Matory, J. Lorand. 2008. "The Illusion of Isolation: The Gullah/Geechees and the Political Economy of African Culture in the Americas." *Comparative Studies in Society and History* 50, no. 4 (October): 949–80.

Occupational Safety and Health Administration. n.d. "Commercial Fishing: Fall Protection Fishing Safety Fact Sheet." Accessed August 31, 2023. https://www.osha.gov/sites/default/files/publications/fallprotectionsafety-commercialfishing-factsheet.pdf.

Parsons, Michelle. 2022. "Thinking About Social Determinants of Health Through the Relationality of Work and Drug Use." *Medical Anthropology Quarterly* 36, no. 2 (February): 272–89.

Pougnet, Richard, Laurence Pougnet, Brice Loddé Loddé, Maria Luisa Canals-Pol, Dominique Jegaden, David Lucas, and Jean-Dominique Dewitte. "Cardiovascular Risk Factors in Seamen and Fishermen: Review of Literature." *International Maritime Health* 64, no. 3 (September): 107–13.

Robertson, Steve. 2007. *Understanding Men and Health: Masculinities, Identity, and Well-Being.* Maidenhead: Open University Press.

Scheper-Hughes, Nancy, and Margaret Locke. 1987. "The Mindful Body. A Prolegomenon to Future Work in Medical Anthropology." *Medical Anthropology Quarterly* 1, no. 1 (March): 6–41.

Segal, Lynne. 1990. *Slow Motion: Changing Masculinities, Changing Men.* New Brunswick: Rutgers University Press.

Soleo, Leonardo, Emanuele Cannizzaro, Piero Lovreglio, Antonella Basso, Maria Nicolá D'Errico, and Enrico Pira. 2013. "Protocols for the Health Surveillance of Fisherman." *Giornale Italiano di Medicina del Lavoro Ergonomia* 35, no. 4 (October-December): 222–26.

Sonvisen, Signe Annie, Trine M. Thorvaldsen, and Jahn Petter Johnsen. 2017. "Governing the Fisher Body—Safety as Body-Politics and Fisheries Governance." *Maritime Studies* 16, no. 9 (July): 29–39.

Sweeney Tookes, Jennifer, Peggy Barlett, and Tracy Yandle. 2018. "The Case for Local and Sustainable Seafood: A Georgia Example." *The Journal of Culture, Agriculture, Food, and the Environment* 40, no. 1 (June): 55–64.

United States Census Bureau. n.d. "County Poverty Rate for the United States: 2013–2017." Accessed August 31, 2023. https://www.census.gov/library/visualizations/2018/comm/acs-5yr-poverty-all-counties.html.

United States Government Accountability Office. 2022. "Coast Guard: Additional Actions Needed to Improve Commercial Fishing Vessel Safety Efforts." Accessed August 31, 2023. https://www.gao.gov/products/gao-23-105289.

Walter, Nicholas, Philippe Bourgois, and H. Margarita Loinaz. 2002. "Masculinity and Undocumented Labor Migration: Injured Latino Day Laborers in San Francisco." *Social Science and Medicine* 59 no. 6: 1159–68.

World Health Organization. 2023. "Social Determinants of Health." Accessed August 31, 2023. https://www.who.int/health-topics/social-determinants-of-health#tab=tab_1.

Yandle, Tracy, Jennifer Sweeney Tookes, and Gina Shamshak. 2019. "Federal Regulatory Impact on Southeastern Crews and Processor Employees: A Pilot Study." Project Report to Funder: *National Marine Fisheries Service's Marine Fisheries Initiative* (MARFIN).

Chapter 6

"Just for Comfort"

Cultural Imaginaries about Extended Breast/Chestfeeding among Medical and Legal Authorities in the United States

Cassandra White

> "You can stop nursing now. It's just for comfort at this point anyway."
>
> "The milk you're producing has no nutritional value, so you should go ahead and wean."
>
> "You're just doing it for yourself at this point."
>
> "Go cold turkey today!"

The above are common unsolicited comments that people who practice "extended" breast/chestfeeding (which I primarily refer to as EN—extended nursing—in this chapter) in the United States hear from others, including family members, friends, colleagues, daycare operators, healthcare professionals, and representatives of the legal system. Many people who nurse children beyond infancy and toddlerhood are told by others that they are doing it "just for comfort," referring to the misconception that human milk magically loses all nutritional value after a certain time and that beyond that time, EN is about coddling children and/or meeting the needs of self-serving adults and that EN can cause physical or psychological problems. Comments and actions associated with urging or mandating people to wean their children before they are ready can cause harm and distress, particularly when they come from people in positions of power or authority, as with healthcare professionals or representatives of the legal system, and can serve to erode the bodily autonomy of both parent and child. Such comments reflect a neoliberal ethos, bolstered by historical factors that led to EN becoming "out of place" in US society and by larger societal pressures and systems in place, such as limited or nonexistent parental leave and inflexible work policies that make it challenging to carry out gentle weaning of child-led weaning. This ethos and portrayal of EN as "out of place" discourages physicians, dentists, attorneys, judges, and others who wield authoritative knowledge from seeking information that might counter their implicit, deeply ingrained biases or that might fill in their knowledge gaps related to EN.

In the United States, parenting practices that include both nursing for what is considered an "extended" time and child-led or gentle weaning of children, are often seen to be abnormal, strange, disgusting, harmful, and even abusive. There are many popular cultural imaginaries, with no scientific basis, about appropriate weaning times that have emerged primarily after the widespread introduction of commercial formula, so that a few generations of people in the United States have had little exposure to seeing children who can walk or talk but who also drink milk from a parent or caregiver's body. Often these imaginaries are linked to developmental milestones (for example, the eruption of teeth, first words, the ability to walk, talk, reach for a breast, etc.), which coincide with beliefs about how a child's maturation should be linked to independence and "no longer needing" either human milk or the close body contact with the parent that breastfeeding/chestfeeding entails.

In this chapter, after providing a brief background of how EN came to be highly stigmatized in the United States, I give examples from ethnographic research with caregivers/parents who practice EN of how medical and legal professionals and institutions wield power, often based on popular imaginaries that nonetheless are presented as authoritative knowledge, to control and coerce caregivers to wean their children abruptly and before they are ready, which can have potential negative emotional, psychological, and physical consequences for both parents and children. Many healthcare professionals have only minimal knowledge about EN and often encourage or mandate weaning when it is not medically necessary. Pediatric dentists in particular can exert authority over parents, shaming them for nursing children to sleep even though the data on the relationship of breast milk to dental caries suggests that multiple factors can be involved in the development of dental problems. Legal issues related to EN are perhaps the biggest threat to the agency and autonomy of children and lactating caregivers in custody cases and in cases where the nursing parent faces time in jail or prison. Biomedical professionals and representatives of the legal system can chip away at the bodily autonomy of people who practice EN and of their children, and they diminish the agency that is often already constrained by pressure from family and work-related pressures to wean. Racial identity, income, education, gender identity, and many other intersecting factors also come into play in terms of the different forms of capital that parents/caregivers can draw on to resist these external threats to their parenting decisions. The construction of EN as a taboo or problematic caregiving practice in the United States facilitates the policing of bodies of people who are already marginalized in different ways because of their age and gender identities (including children and caregivers who are primarily cisgender women, nonbinary people assigned female at birth, and transgender men) in a way that fits into a neoliberal definition of productivity.

ETHNOGRAPHIC PERSPECTIVES ON EXPERIENCES OF EN IN THE UNITED STATES

My interest in this topic emerged during the five years and about three months that I nursed my son. I had somewhat casually committed to an attachment parenting style that included child-led weaning, but I did not anticipate how long and how challenging of a commitment this could be; I expected child-led weaning to happen between ages 2–4, which is what most parenting books suggested. Even when my son stopped nursing, a few months after his fifth birthday, weaning was not 100 percent child-led but a combination of strategies so that he would fall asleep on his own and be too distracted during the day to ask for milk. The intense and interesting experience of these years of nursing my son, during which I lacked a shared community with whom to discuss the challenges of EN, inspired a decade of IRB-approved digital ethnographic research, primarily on social media support groups for EN, parenting groups, breast/chestfeeding pages and accounts on Facebook (primarily), Instagram, TikTok, and Reddit. This research involved extensive participation in public and private groups and included reaching out frequently via private messaging to gain consent to use a paraphrased version of a post or comment or to gather additional information about a post or comment. In addition, I recruited a small number of people who had practiced EN for two years or more for in-depth in-person or virtual interviews through both convenience sampling and through social media. I conducted five interviews in 2017, and seven in 2022–2023, with the latter set giving an interesting perspective on EN during the COVID-19 pandemic. While interview questions were initially designed around questions and themes that emerged during my own experience with EN, with participant observation in digital spaces, I identified new themes that emerged that differed from my own experiences as a white, middle-class anthropologist, and I was able to explore a wider range of topics related to EN in the United States.

A NOTE ON TERMINOLOGY

The terminology I use in discussing this work has evolved over time, which is one advantage of a longer-term study. I acknowledge that "extended" is an entirely relative term when it comes to nursing a child. For the study, I defined "extended" as "2 years or more," which correlates to a World Health Organization recommendation, although it was only in 2022 that the American Academy of Pediatrics updated their recommendations to match those of the WHO (Meek et al. 2022, 4), including a statement that they support "continued breastfeeding along with appropriate complementary foods introduced at about 6 months, as long as mutually desired by mother and child for 2 years or beyond." The main criterion for participation in in-depth interviews or private discussions for which people had given consent for me to use in this study was nursing a child from the body for two years or more, but on social media sites, there was a wide range of people who had self-identified as practicing EN but who had not reached the two-year mark but still experienced stigma associated the nursing their children longer than others felt was necessary or normal.

I initially used the terms "women" and "breastfeeding" to discuss this topic, but through in-depth interviews and digital ethnography, I learned more about the experiences of people who nursed their children but did not identify as cisgender women. People who were assigned female at birth but who identify as nonbinary or as trans men can also feed children from their breasts. Humans of all gender identities have breasts and milk ducts, though the development of the latter is hormone-dependent, so that most cisgender men's milk ducts are underdeveloped; there are known cases in which people who were assigned male at birth can lactate and can produce milk that contains nutritional value similar to that of cisgender women or trans or nonbinary men who were assigned female at birth (Kolski et al. 1981). "Chestfeeding" is often the preferred term today for people for whom the term "breasts" is associated with dysphoria and/or sexualization (Bartick et al. 2021). In presenting this research, I use breast/chestfeeding or the abbreviation EN (extended nursing), which remove suggestions of gender identity of the lactating caregiver. In observations in virtual spaces and in individual interviews, I have focused on primarily on people who also identify as a parent to a child or children to whom they have fed milk from their bodies.

STIGMA, AUTONOMY, AND EN IN THE UNITED STATES

Breast/chestfeeding children beyond infancy and often beyond the toddler stage was common for most of human and hominid prehistory (Dettwyler 1995; Stuart-Macadam 1995); however, the emergence of stratified societies and particularly shifts in labor have greatly altered nursing practices, so that it is overly simplistic to say that all or most babies were nursed for several years or were allowed to wean themselves before the introduction of commercial formula. In the US context historically, chattel slavery greatly impacted nursing practices and had long-lasting effects on how nursing a child from the breast was perceived in the African American community, as many enslaved people were separated from their biological children or served as wet nurses for white children, limiting the time they could spend nursing and caring for their own children (Freeman 2020). The industrial revolution and the rise of global capitalism also led many working-class families to seek wet nurses (often among women from more "destitute" families) so that birthing adults in a family could return to work and not lose wages (Stevens et al. 2009). Foucault (1995, 160), in *Discipline and Punish*, that the "observed new techniques of power" that corresponded with the rise of capitalism included "a new way of administering time and making it useful," while also redefining usefulness and productivity.

Although the seeds of a neoliberal ethos as it relates to the breast/chestfeeding relationship were being planted during the colonial era, the commercial formula and baby food industries, starting in the late nineteenth century but reaching global distribution in the twentieth century, had the most significant impact on making bottle and formula-feeding the norm. Thulier (2009, 90), in a historical retrospective of breastfeeding in the United States, compared data on breastfeeding throughout the twentieth century. Between the 1930s and 1970, the percentage of children who were still being breastfed after three months dropped from 70 percent to just 8 percent; by 1970, only 28 percent of infants were ever breastfed. Although there were subsequent global and national health campaigns to encourage nursing, the near disappearance of the practice of nursing a child even beyond infancy during these decades created a distance that makes it seem strange and anomalous. Increased sexualization of women's breasts in the second half of the twentieth century further contributed to ideas that EN was an overtly sexual act that could be psychologically damaging to children. As the highlighting of women's breasts as objects of sexual desire increased, the expectation that breasts that were feeding a human child needed to be covered up was amplified (Zaikman and Houlihan 2022). Public breast/chestfeeding and EN in particular came to be seen in the United States as practices that were relegated to the "other"—to non-Western, rural cultures or foraging societies. In Mary Douglas's schema (1966) for explaining why some behaviors, objects, or practices are taboo or stigmatized, things that fall outside of established cultural categories are seen as taboo and often symbolically "unclean," which can also render things to seen as not only disgusting but dangerous. Early weaning from the breast and supplementation with formula feeding, or formula feeding alone, became normative and came to seem "natural" to many people in the United States. Bourdieu's conception of *doxa* is also useful to explain that when practices and beliefs are accepted as normal and are thus seen as "self-evident and undisputed" (Bourdieu 1992, 164). Doxa also serve to uphold societal structures, so they are difficult to contest or resist.

As EN became taboo, a number of cultural imaginaries developed around the practice. Many imaginaries, drawing on Charles Taylor's understanding of the term (2004) are popular beliefs that seem to draw on scientific thinking but that have little to no basis in science. The most common cultural imaginaries about when to wean are often linked to developmental milestones, though there is no scientific evidence that any of these milestones necessitate weaning or are "natural" times for weaning in humans or nonhuman primates. For example: "Once a child develops teeth, they should be weaned," or "If a child can ask for milk, they are too old to be nursing." Both of these milestones (eruption of teeth and first words) are seemingly nonsensically linked to the need to wean a child in the popular imagination; infants develop teeth fairly early, and some are born with teeth, which have little to do with being able to nurse a child; many children can communicate through either signs or words that they want milk before they are a year old. These statements are an indication that in the cultural imaginary, weaning and maturity are linked in such a way that it is hard for people to conceive that children's intellectual, social, physical, and emotional development is not impeded by breast/chestfeeding. The cultural embodiment of neoliberal values that require children to develop into independent and self-actualized beings quickly and that require a return to work for their parents both creates and reinforces the idea that a child who can walk or talk is "too old" to be nursing.

Foucault's concept of biopower (1978) is also useful for thinking about how control is exerted by capitalist and neoliberal forces that encourage early weaning or that make EN and child-led weaning difficult, though not impossible, and that make EN subject to shame and stigma if it is known about by or visible to others. EN has been constructed as delaying the development not only of the child as the "ideal neoliberal subject" (Moss and Roberts-Homes 2021:2) but of the breast/chestfeeding parent whose economic productivity is potentially decreased. Many parents who practice EN come to realize that being "subjected to a field of visibility," as Foucault (1995, 202) described in writing about the power of Bentham's panopticon, increases vulnerability and makes resistance to societal pressures to wean more difficult. Goffman (1963, 54) wrote that some stigmatizing attributes "are so easily concealed that they figured very little in the individual's relation to strangers and mere acquaintances." Most of the caregivers I interviewed in in-depth interviews talked about only disclosing that they were still nursing after toddlerhood in selected contexts so as to avoid negative comments or scrutiny. In public settings, concealment can require self-policing and policing of children's words and actions in terms of how they ask for milk, whether the lactating parent uses a cover or cloth while nursing, or whether they are allowed to pull on the lactating parent's clothing or unbutton their shirt; setting boundaries on children's nursing behaviors becomes easier as children develop more complex communication skills, though this depends on the child. There are times, though, when concealment of EN becomes impossible, as in cases of the need for biomedical care or treatment (for the child or parent) or in some legal situations, in which parenting practices become more visible and thus subject to the gaze of biomedical or legal authorities.

AUTHORITATIVE IMAGINARIES

Despite recommendations that have been set and promoted by respected global and national health organization about breast/chestfeeding and EN, those trained in medical and legal fields often retain biases from their personal experiences and backgrounds and can hold explanatory models of health, illness, and the body that do not match scientific explanatory models (McCombie 1999; Kuhns 2012). In the absence of firsthand experience of or education about EN, legal professionals in the United States also bring cultural imaginaries about EN to their work in the court system. Implicit racial and gender bias is well-documented in the US legal system (Kang et al. 2011), which can further complicate outcomes related to cases involving EN. Below I give some examples of my interlocutors' encounters with biomedical and legal systems in the United States.

The Biomedical Encounter and EN

In online EN communities, there is almost daily mention of pressure from healthcare professionals to wean. Most posts of this nature are followed by a few to sometimes hundreds of comments of support, and many people will share websites and peer-reviewed articles, with the suggestion that they share this information with the healthcare professional in question. To begin this section, I highlight the story of one of my in-depth interviewees here. All names used here are pseudonyms. Deanna (a pseudonym) identifies as multiracial (her mother is white and father is African American). In early 2020, Deanna private messaged me after seeing a post I made about my research on a Facebook group. She told me that her son had recently turned two, and she said she started to get a lot of flak about nursing. "Everyone is horrified—even my very educated and forward-thinking family and my pediatrician." She said that when the pediatrician found out that Deanna was breastfeeding, "she said, 'Oh no! Quit that now, he doesn't need it. Go cold turkey today!! But that was six months ago,' when Deanna's son was just eighteen months old. 'I shudder to think what she would say now.' Deanna herself, who has a bachelor's degree and has worked in public health research contexts, felt that this advice was problematic, so she sought out a nonprofit lactation consultant, who validated Deanna on her decision to continue nursing, as I did when we communicated. Deanna described how the pediatrician's words reinforced pressure that was coming from her mother to wean: "As I recall, my mother was in the room when the pediatrician was telling me to go cold turkey ASAP. And she was nodding like 'see?' It was/is infuriating. From what I've read, that's not good for anyone. The doctor said that it was me who wasn't ready to wean."

As a recognized source of authority, this pediatrician's stance, which included the very common popular imaginary that people practicing EN are doing it "for themselves" (a belief that is often discussed as absurd on support groups, given the challenges involved), reinforced Deanna's mother's position, creating more issues for Deanna and further subverting Deanna's autonomy in decision-making. Deanna also said: "We also co-slept for about a year/ year and a half. And again, you'd think I beat him the way folks reacted. Secretly I still lay next to him and rub his back until he sleeps. I'm a rebel." Pediatricians frequently ask about sleeping arrangements, and the American Academy of Pediatrics hard line on co-sleeping (AAP 2022) makes it less likely that nursing will continue for more than a few months; EN parents, many of whom co-sleep at some point, may be less likely to reveal their sleeping arrangements to healthcare professionals. While there are dangers to bedsharing with an infant, most infant deaths have been linked to bedding or other hazardous sleeping arrangement and overlaying or to intoxication on the part of a parent; these are real dangers in many US households, and the AAP has chosen to strongly suggest that infants sleep separately from adults in their own crib, though in the same room. Breast/chestfeeding is correlated with a lower risk of sudden infant death syndrome, but biological anthropologist James McKenna has suggested that bedsharing/co-sleeping, which is more common among parents who nurse, could be the protective variable in preventing SIDS (McKenna and McDade 2005; McKenna et al. 2007).

Deanna was able to resist attempts by her son's pediatrician to compel her to wean her son in part because she had access to social and cultural capital, including online networks and her own education and public health experience, despite the fact that siblings and other family members weaned their children much earlier, at "six or eight months," so she did not have allies within the family. Deanna did repeat the imaginary that she had been told by others, it was "only for comfort," but she also saw this as a positive thing: "It helps him sleep and calm down after he's hurt. But I'm treated like I'm doing him some disservice at this age. I feel like there's some clock looming over us and I'd better wean him now even if I'm not sure that he's ready."

In 2022, I arranged an in-depth virtual interview with Deanna, then in her early forties. She said weaned her son at 3.5 years. In this interview, she reflected on her experience with physicians when her son was still nursing, because he when he was very little, she was able to witness how beneficial breastfeeding was to him. He suffered a serious injury as an infant, and she said, "We would not have made it through if he didn't get to nurse. And, I mean that for, like, the nutrition and the emotional side of that, you know," which is why, she said, "I was kind of scratching my head" at the medical community's response.

Melissa, a white woman (in her early 40s when I interviewed her in 2022), had practiced EN with four children and tandem nursed throughout the pandemic. She said that while she was not pressured to wean by physicians, "there were times when I wanted to do something for my own health, like go on a different medication, and then I couldn't because of breastfeeding. I want to say there were some times where I thought, 'well, I don't think that's really true from my research, but you're the doctor.'"

On social media support groups, it is also common to see posts in which physicians assume that certain medications cannot be taken by lactating parents but have not done any research to see if that is truly the case. I was in touch with Camila, a Black and Latina mom in her 20s, after I saw a post she made about being compelled in wean her child because of a medication she later found out was not, in fact, contraindicated in breast/chestfeeding; by the time she found this out, her milk supply had diminished, and she was struggling to relactate.

While there are medications and courses of treatment that are unsafe for lactating parents to take because of the risks to their nursing children, according to the Mayo Clinic (2022), most are safe, including several antidepressants, steroids, and many other medications. Physicians might also make recommendations without distinguishing infants from children two and over, for whom the small amount of a medication that might enter breast milk will be less of a risk. It is fairly simple for healthcare professionals to find links to peer-reviewed articles or websites from respected biomedical authorities that give information about medications or procedures that are contraindicated for nursing parents, but the onus is often on the parent to access and bring information to the clinic. In some cases, nursing parents feel coerced into making a choice between weaning before they are ready (as in Camila's case) or not taking a medication that could improve their health and well-being (as Melissa did).

The most frequent concerns about EN, based on comments and searches I have done within support groups on Facebook, are expressed by pediatric dentists. From a scientific perspective, a cause-effect relationship between EN and dental problems, especially with night nursing, is quite complicated, and most dentists seem to be unaware of the nuances. Some children who nurse throughout the night for years (including my child) never get cavities or have any other dental problems. In support groups, there are many testimonies of long-term night nursing with no cavities as well as other possible culprits for cavities (lip ties, tongue ties, mouth breathing, child's diet of solid foods or sugary drinks, genetics, enamel hypoplasia, and more). However, when nursing children do present with a cavity or multiple cavities, dentists can be quick to suggest that night nursing is the sole cause and that weaning, at least night weaning (arguably the most difficult to wean toddlers and older children from once it has been established), is the only and "easiest" solution, though in practice, it is quite difficult and can feel devastating to nursing parents and children.

Members of online support groups for EN relate stories of pediatric dentists who suggest not only night weaning but fairly drastic approaches to cavities in nursing children, such as hospital-based surgical removal of teeth, root canals, and intensive fluoride treatments. Dentists often tell parents that it is caused by the pooling of breast milk in the mouth/sleeping with this pooled milk against the teeth, although there is evidence (Ribeiro and Ribeiro 2004, whose work is cited in a publication of the American Dental Association by Seale et al. 2013:148) that "the biomechanics of breastfeeding differ from those of bottle feeding, with the result being that breast milk is expressed into the soft palate and swallowed."

"I feel so guilty" was a common sentiment on posts about this, and "I feel like a terrible parent." These sentiments are reinforced by the language of dental healthcare professionals, who will often say that night nursing "ruins" children's teeth in the same way that formula might in what's called "bottle rot" or "baby bottle tooth decay." This also results in parents who practice night nursing to second-guess their decisions about EN. The visible nature of cavities and the fears of the negative health consequences that can arise also create additional pressures to wean from family members who were unsupportive of EN in the first place.

The most helpful comments in support groups, I believe, are those that discuss examples of dentists who were better informed and who had strategies for effective interventions that limit progression of tooth decay while allowing night nursing to continue. Some dentists suggest "wiping teeth" after the last feeding, which many caregivers felt was a somewhat impractical suggestion, as with children who nurse to sleep, there is almost no way to do this without waking them up, and the reality is that night nursing can take place multiple times in a night in a co-sleeping situation. Other interventions discussed include use of fluoride or silver nitrate treatments and xylitol-based toothpastes.

It is clear from posts and comments that finding a solution that does not include abrupt weaning from night nursing requires significant intellectual and emotional labor and time, which can involve seeking a dentist who is more familiar with the complex factors that can cause dental problems in young children or doing research online or through support groups and becoming an "expert" on the topic themselves. In one support group post, it was mentioned that a dentist said that infant/child feeding with human milk is generally not discussed as part of their training. A 2019 survey of early-career dentists in the UK indicated that the majority of "early-career" dentists received very little training about breast/chestfeeding (Polglass et al.), though I have not located similar studies in the US context.

In online support groups, there were also examples of posts that documented positive experiences with biomedical providers. Often this happened because a healthcare professional themselves had practiced EN with their own child or children. Posts from parents practicing EN who describe being shamed and urged to stop nursing by healthcare professionals were much more common than positive anecdotes, however. For Deanna, her son's pediatrician's statements about weaning seemed to be based entirely on cultural imaginaries about "natural" or "normal" times to wean. Melissa and Camila's experiences represent more of a knowledge gap on the part of physicians about whether certain medications were safe for nursing parents. These knowledge gaps about EN, night nursing, and breast/chestfeeding in general seem to be pervasive and highlight the importance of including more information about these topics in medical and dental school curricula.

Legal Issues

In legal cases, the authority and power of the courts can be difficult to counter, even for parents/caregivers with significant social and cultural capital. Legal issues that people wrote about and sought advice for on social media groups alerted me to issues that I had not previously considered when I began this research. My only encounters with the legal system when I was practicing

EN were calls for jury duty. I assumed it would be easy for nursing parents to defer their service if there were no private spaces to pump milk; in my case it was easy, but my impression was that the clerk I spoke to each time had very little knowledge about breast/chestfeeding at all or about EN and allowed me to defer because I asked the right questions about services that were available to me. This was also in a relatively progressive county (Dekalb County, Georgia), but since then, on local parenting groups, I have observed many complaints about jury duty being mandated for someone who is still nursing an infant or child.

On social media support groups for EN, the most common legal issue that people ask questions about (or just seek moral support) arise in cases of separation and divorce. In custody cases, it is not just legal authorities who play a part in making decisions that force the child to be weaned. Generally, the other parent or guardian plays a large role in this; if the other parent is supportive of EN, typically there is less of an issue, and compromises on time spent with each parent can work out well. In contrast, when the non-nursing parent is unsupportive of EN, they can often use the legal system to their advantage.

One of my participants in in-depth interviews, Alyssa, a white woman and graduate student who was in her twenties when I first interviewed her for this research in 2017 and who practiced child-led weaning with her children, kept in touch with me and told me about issues related to nursing, domestic violence, and custody for a child she had a few years later; in 2022, she was living in a state where the rights of the biological fathers to access to their children was typically upheld by judges. Often this includes approving custody arrangements in which both parents share significant time with a child, including overnight visits, which can be particularly difficult when a child is still nursing. In her case, despite a history of domestic violence and lack of involvement by the father, and despite this child being under two and still nursing, the court had granted him rights to overnights, an order which she fought. She talked to me about the case when it was ongoing: "If I'm in the top 2 percent most educated women in the world and have a family that can send me 10K for attorneys, and I still can't escape this, then what hope is there for anyone?" In the end, through extensive self-advocacy and her own ability to understand and to research options led to a positive outcome in which she gained full custody and decided after this to dedicate her own work and research to helping others in similar situations.

I communicated with several women through private messaging who had less favorable outcomes and were being compelled to wean before they were ready; some were parents practicing EN who requested an "expert letter," which I have sent to several parents after I mentioned this in comments on EN support groups. Anthropologist Katherine Dettwyler also crafted a court letter that she posted to her website (Dettwyler 2015) but posted that in retirement, she could no longer send signed letters. I shared my version of a court letter with over a dozen women on Facebook support groups for EN. I point out, in the letter, that prioritizing the needs of children who are still nursing does not have to detract from the relationship with the non-lactating parent if they are able to be patient and flexible. Through sharing the letter, I had a chance to learn about several lengthy custody battles in from people around the United States (and also the UK); in general, the courts have a great deal of power to order an abrupt end to breastfeeding/chestfeeding, especially for people practicing EN, though this still regularly occurs with infants who are nursing as well. I also received consent to share a modified version of some of their stories.

Shelly, a white woman with whom I exchanged several messages over a two-year period, was practicing EN with her child and wanted to continue after a divorce from her husband. A guardian ad litem was assigned to her child, which is a person who is assigned by the courts to advise on what is in the best interests of the child. Shelly told me: "the guardian ad litem assigned to my kid is pushing me to wean. I am so sad. I know my son is going through so much and weaning him at such a difficult time (divorce, starting daycare, etc.) is really not being child-centric." Several months later, she was issued a court order to "cease and desist" from both breastfeeding and co-sleeping. Shelly messaged that "this [EN] is what is seen as an anomaly and problem, vs. the emotional and psychological abuse" and evidence of other forms of violence from her ex-husband. She said that EN was seen as something that was being used by the courts to question her fitness as a mom. "And a good mom is all I want to be to my son," she said. As in Alyssa's case, Shelly mobilized different resources to fight this, including accessing resources through Facebook private support groups; in addition to letters I prepared, she had a letter from a pediatrician who was supportive of EN. She also fired her lawyer; ultimately the court order was not upheld, despite urging from the guardian ad litem, but the process for her case is ongoing.

Another legal issue related to EN that I have come across on social media posts is jail or prison time that also strips lactating parents and children of autonomy by physically separating them. In a few posts, people have brought up concerns about short jail sentences, often for nonviolent offenses, in which no attention or assistance is given to nursing mothers, who risk infections (especially mastitis) if unable to pump or express their milk; this also can cause severe distress for young children. This is a larger issue that relates to breast/chestfeeding in general and also raises (or answers) questions about whether or not the courts have the best interests of infants and children in mind when parents are sentenced to serve time away from their children. Although the National Commission on Correctional Healthcare has a list of best practices regarding lactating caregivers who are incarcerated (including accommodations for pumping and for frequent visits), there are only a handful of nursery programs in US prisons, but they are for parents of nursing infants (NCCHC 2023; Thorne 2022). Another population that is typically overlooked and rendered virtually invisible are parents who are incarcerated in immigrant detention facilities; Rabin (2008, 717) highlights documented cases of breastfeeding mothers being separated from their children, including one case in which a woman was detained at Eloy Detention Center in Arizona "without access to a breast pump to relieve and maintain her milk supply; she was unable to continue breastfeeding upon release." Gender identity can add an additional layer of risk of juridical challenges to parental fitness, particularly in US states where discriminatory laws have been passed regarding the expression of trans and nonbinary identities. Social media platforms, particularly Facebook videos, Instagram reels, and TikTok videos, are spaces where some trans and nonbinary people are open about nursing their infants and children in a form of visibility that has the potential to normalize the practice but simultaneously fuels moral panic that can perpetuate societal stigma and cultural imaginaries about both trans identity and breast/chestfeeding.

Perhaps even more than in the biomedical field, cultural imaginaries that "seem" to reflect "traditional values," are slow to change, particularly when they serve to maintain systems that benefit those in power. Amy, who I interviewed in 2022, practiced EN with both of her children; she is a white, middle-upper-class attorney who also became a La Leche League leader. She said that "most male judges are over 50, maybe they have some memories of their wives breastfeeding, but basically probably have negative associations" with it in general, so misconceptions and knowledge gaps about EN are common. Her experience with EN and efforts to educate herself, in part due to a constant struggle with her mother-in-law about weaning, also had an impact on her husband, who, while serving as a judge, implemented accommodations for nursing parents when they were serving jury duty. Without the personal experience of practicing or living with someone who practiced EN, most people in positions of authority in the court system will be unaware of how cultural imaginaries and biases shape decisions related to people practicing EN.

A PATH TO RENORMALIZATION OF EN?

Douglas (1966, 40) noted that cultural categories provide a "pattern in which ideas and values are tidily ordered," and because these categories are "public matters," they "cannot be easily subject to revision." The cultural imaginaries that have developed around EN and child-led weaning persist and may take many years to shift at a societal level. The research presented in this chapter on the experiences of people who practice EN demonstrates that they are vulnerable in interactions with healthcare and legal professionals and systems that retain biases and misconceptions about EN, thus threatening not only the breast/chestfeeding relationship but the rights of lactating caregivers to care for their children altogether. Incorporation of information about EN in particular in law, medical, dental, and public health curricula is important in the future in terms of decreasing the knowledge gaps that allow people in positions of authority to erode parental and child autonomy.

Even with increased education about the practice, reconstructing EN as a normal and acceptable practice may be difficult in a neoliberal economy. Moore and Robinson (2016) suggested that in the contemporary workplace, characterized by "precarity, austerity, intense competition for jobs and anxieties with robots and other machines as well as, themselves replaceable, humans, workers are compelled to squeeze every last drop of labour-power from their bodies" (2775). I thought this was an apt metaphor, if unintentional on the authors' parts, for how EN is constructed as "unproductive"; if "every last drop" of a person's labor is to be invested in paid labor, what are the chances that a society based on neoliberal values would provide the support for lactating caregivers to offer milk on demand and to take a more relaxed approach to weaning? Smith (2013), in discussing the tension between feminist arguments that breast/chestfeeding is constraining for women and breastfeeding advocates position that it can be liberating, wrote: "Society makes choices about when, where, and to what extent it will and will not value, recognize, and adjust to the needs of bodies. The dividing line may arise from benign neglect, from ignorance, or from an interest in creating or preserving particular power structures."

Flexible work policies could facilitate EN for those who want to practice it. Some of my interlocutors mentioned work-from-home policies during the pandemic that made on-demand nursing easier and made it easier to "hide" the fact that they were practicing EN, but they still had to keep up with their work responsibilities along with full-time childcare at home. In addition, social class and employment type dictates which lactating parents were able to work remotely during the pandemic or who can take advantage of flexible work policies in general. The United States is still very far from enacting policies that would allow EN and child-led weaning to work well for parents across different demographics to the point where EN could be normalized. The United States is still one of the only countries in the world with zero weeks that are federally mandated for paid parental leave of any type, although some individual states have paid leave policies. In 2021, among the 186 countries with paid maternity leave policies, the average duration is

29 weeks; among the 109 countries with paternity leave, the average time is 16 weeks (Miller 2021).

Labor and leave policies and recommendations by nationally-recognized medical and legal professional associations are vital for normalization of EN to occur, but cultural imaginaries about EN can persist even with these policies in place. Andrews's (2022) research in Norway, which has a generous policy for parental leave, demonstrates that while breast/ chestfeeding itself is normalized and expected, there is a strong stigma against weaning "too late." As in the United States (but to an even greater degree in Norway), parents who are unable to initiate nursing, who prefer to bottle-feed, or who wean "too early" are also subjected to stigma and shame. Andrews observed that "in both cases, mothers have been accused of giving priority to their own needs rather than putting their child's health and well-being first" (2022, 66). This is a good example of how biopower can operate to coerce health-related and parenting behaviors. I would like to emphasize that while normalization of EN is important to protect people and their children from biomedical and legislative interventions, EN does not have to become an expectation or a standard for parenting; in my research, the parents who practice EN primarily hoped that it could be a choice that is free from stigma.

Although the burden of normalization of EN should not reside with people who practice it, those who are comfortable being open with this practice and who have the social and cultural capital to be advocates for themselves and others may make an impact in terms of shifting cultural dialogues about this practice. Several of the participants in the in-depth interviews I conducted for this study sought additional education or professional training after their children were weaned or while they were still nursing because they wanted to help other parents with issues related to EN and breast/chestfeeding initiation in general. Over the last decade, I have observed many examples of how people who practice EN access different social media groups to increase the visibility of EN (on more public-facing social media sites like TikTok), to support others practicing EN, and to share information and resources. This kind of mutual aid allows people who practice EN to resist societal pressures and contest biomedical and legal authority in innovative ways so that they may retain some say in feeding and weaning decisions and can, in turn, renormalize EN.

REFERENCES CITED

AAP (American Academy of Pediatrics). 2022. "American Academy of Pediatrics Updates Safe Sleep Recommendations: Back is Best." Accessed August 21,

2023. https://www.aap.org/en/news-room/news-releases/aap/2022/american-academy-of-pediatrics-updates-safe-sleep-recommendations-back-is-best/.

Andrews, Therese. 2022. "Modern Taboos and Moral Regulations: Mother's Milk in the Symbolic Order." Sociology, Vol. 56(1) 55–71.

Bartick, Melissa, Elizabeth K. Stehel, Sarah L. Calhoun, Lori Feldman-Winter, Deena Zimmerman, Lawrence Noble, Casey Rosen-Carole, Laura R. Kair, and the Academy of Breastfeeding Medicine. 2021. "Academy of Breastfeeding Medicine Position Statement and Guideline: infant feeding and lactation-related language and gender." *Breastfeeding Medicine* 16, no. 8: 587–90.

Bourdieu, Pierre. 1992. *Outline of a Theory of Practice*. Translated by Richard Nice. New York: Cambridge University Press.

Dettwyler, Katherine A. 1995. "A Time to Wean: The Hominid for the Natural Age of Weaning in Modern Human Populations. In *Breastfeeding: Biocultural Perspectives*, edited by Patricia Stuart-Macadam and Katherine A. Dettwyler, 39–73. New York: Aldine de Gruyter.

———. 2015. "Inside the Mind of Kathy Dettwyler," Accessed August 13, 2023. http://kathydettwyler.weebly.com/2015-court-letter.html.

Douglas, Mary. 1966. *Purity and Danger: An Analysis of Concepts of Purity and Taboo*. New York: Routledge.

Foucault, Michel. 1978. *The History of Sexuality, Vol. 1: An Introduction*. Translation by Robert Hurley. New York: Pantheon Books.

———. 1995. *Discipline and Punish: The Birth of the Prison*. Translated by Alan Sheridan. New York: Vintage Books.

Freeman, Andrea. 2020. *Skimmed: Breastfeeding, Race, and Injustice*. Stanford: Stanford University Press.

Goffman, E. (1963). *Stigma: Notes on the Management of Spoiled Identity*. Hoboken, NJ: Prentice Hall.

Kang, Jerry, Mark Bennett, Devon Carbado, Pam Casey, Nilanjana Dasgupta, David Faigman, Rachel Godsil, Anthony G. Greenwald, Justin Levinson, Jennifer Mnookin. 2012. "Implicit bias in the courtroom." *UCLA Law Review*. 59: 1124–86.

Kuhns, Kristin. 2012. "What's to Know? Navigating Knowledge Gaps of Hansen's Disease in the U.S." MA thesis, Georgia State University. https://scholarworks.gsu.edu/anthro_theses/66/.

Kulski, J. K., P. E. Hartmann, and D. H. Gutteridge. 1981. 'Composition of Breast Fluid of a Man with Galactorrhea and Hyperprolactinaemia." *The Journal of Clinical Endocrinology & Metabolism* 52, no. 3: 581–82. https://doi.org/10.1210/jcem-52-3-581.

Mayo Clinic. 2022. "Breastfeeding and Medications: What's Safe." Accessed August 21, 2023. https://www.mayoclinic.org/healthy-lifestyle/infant-and-toddler-health/in-depth/breastfeeding-and-medications/art-20043975.

McCombie, Susan. 1999. "Folk Flu and Viral Syndrome: An Anthropological Perspective." *Anthropology in Public Health: Bridging Differences in Culture and Society*, edited by Robert Hahn: 27–43.

McKenna, James J., and Thomas McDade. 2005. "Why Babies Should Never Sleep Alone: A Review of the Co-sleeping Controversy in Relation to SIDS, Bedsharing and Breastfeeding." *Paediatric Respiratory Reviews* 6, no. 2: 134–52.

McKenna, James J., Helen L. Ball, and Lee T. Gettler. 2007. "Mother–infant Cosleeping Breastfeeding and Sudden Infant Death Syndrome: What Biological Anthropology has Discovered About Normal Infant Sleep and Pediatric Sleep Medicine." *American Journal of Physical Anthropology: The Official Publication of the American Association of Physical Anthropologists* 134, no. S45: 133–61.

Meek, Joan Younger, Lawrence Noble, and Section on Breastfeeding. 2022. "Policy statement: Breastfeeding and the Use of Human Milk." *Pediatrics* 150, no. 1: e2022057988.

Miller, Claire Cain. 2021. "The World 'Has Found a Way to Do This': The U.S. Lags on Paid Leave." *New York Times*. Accessed August 20, 2023. https://www.nytimes.com/2021/10/25/upshot/paid-leave-democrats.html.

Moore, Phoebe, and Andrew Robinson. 2016. "The Quantified Self: What Counts in the Neoliberal Workplace." *New Media & Society* 18, no.11: 2774–92.

Moss, Peter, and Guy Roberts-Holmes. 2021. "Now is the Time! Confronting Neo-Liberalism in Early Childhood." *Contemporary Issues in Early Childhood*: https://doi.org/10.1177/1463949121995917.

National Commission on Correctional Health Care (NCCHC). 2023. "Breastfeeding in Correctional Settings." Accessed August 15, 2023. https://www.ncchc.org/position-statements/breastfeeding-in-correctional-settings.2023/#:~:text=Research%20has%20shown%20that%20it,breastfeedingg%20(Asiodu%2C%202021).

Polglass, Louisa, Jo Leonardi-Bee, Alexander Morris, and Rachael Murray. 2019. "Promotion of Breastfeeding by Dental Teams: A Survey of Early Career Dentists." *Journal of Health Visiting* 7, no. 1: 24–29. https://doi.org/10.12968/johv.2019.7.1.24.

Rabin, Nina. 2008. "Unseen Prisoners: Women in Immigration Detention Facilities in Arizona." *Georgetown Immigration Law Journal* 23: 695.

Ribeiro NM, Ribeiro MS. 2004. Breastfeeding and Early Childhood Caries: A Critical Review *Jornal da Pediatria* 80, suppl 5.: S199–S210.

Smith, P. H. (2013). Breastfeeding and gender inequality. Journal of Women, Politics & Policy, 34(4), 371–83. https://doi.org/10.1080/1554477X.2013.835682.

Stevens, Emily E., Thelma E. Patrick, and Rita Pickler. 2009. "A History of Infant Feeding." *The Journal of Perinatal Education* 18, no, 2: 32–39.

Stuart-Macadam, Patricia. 1995. "Breastfeeding in Prehistory." In *Breastfeeding: Biocultural Perspectives*, edited by Patricia Stuart-Macadam and Katherine A. Dettwyler, 75–99. New York: Aldine de Gruyter.

Taylor, Charles. 2003. *Modern Social Imaginaries*. Durham, NC: Duke University Press.

Thorne, Kaitlin. 2022. Prison Nurseries Help Incarcerated Mothers Bond, but Options Are Limited. Accessed August 10, 2023. https://www.lpm.org/news/2022-05-30/prison-nurseries-help-incarcerated-mothers-bond-but-options-are-limited.

Thulier, Diane. 2009. "Breastfeeding in America: A History of Influencing Factors." *Journal of Human Lactation* 25, no. 1: 85–94.

Zaikman, Yuliana, and Amy E. Houlihan. 2022. "It's Just a Breast: An Examination of the Effects of Sexualization, Sexism, and Breastfeeding Familiarity on Evaluations of Public Breastfeeding." *BMC Pregnancy and Childbirth* 22, no. 1: 1–16.

Chapter 7

"I Felt Almost Like a Robot Going in That Room"

The Control of Maternal Bodies and Maternal Health in Georgia

Heidi M. Altman and Tobi Oloyede

Women's bodies are the nexus of all aspects of human experience in cultures across the world as the creators of life, the sustainers of new life, and often the caretakers of those passing from this life. In cultural practices that are centered on this view of women's bodies, women are celebrated and venerated as central figures. The status and well-being of women are seen as leading indicators of the health of nations overall (Doepke et al. 2012).

THE MATERNAL HEALTH CRISIS IN THE UNITED STATES AND GEORGIA

If women's well-being is any reflection, the United States is not well. The United States has the worst rates of maternal mortality and morbidity of any of the wealthy Western countries that we consider to be peers. In the United States the rate of maternal mortality is approximately 17 deaths per 100,000 live births. Of the European and English Commonwealth countries, France is next highest with 9 per 100,000 (Tikkanen et al. 2020). And, although this crisis has been apparent since 2013, when the mechanism for reporting maternal deaths changed, and researchers and practitioners in various sectors have focused on making clinical improvements, the numbers are not improving. Even more disturbing, despite nearly a decade of clinical and other interventions, the most recent reporting based on CDC data (Trost et al. 2023) shows that over 85 percent of maternal deaths reviewed were to some degree preventable. This leads us to ask, what lies at the heart of the maternal mortality crisis? If it is not a matter that can be resolved by improving clinical practice, what can be done? Of course, as anthropologists, we look to culture and the practices, beliefs and interactions that enter the delivery room from the lives and experiences of patients and providers.

In the United States, the culture of healthcare is widely variable, especially as it pertains to women's bodies. Access to care is determined by a capricious system that patches together health insurance partially subsidized by large employers, costly private insurance sometimes subsidized by smaller employers, inequitable access to the healthcare marketplace to purchase subsidized care, and federally fully subsidized Medicaid, access to which is widely variable by state. It is nearly impossible to resolve the question of maternal mortality at the federal level, given the myriad conditions in each state—all of which result from political positions on the right to healthcare, the cost of healthcare, and especially the rights of women to control their reproductive lives and experiences. The recent reversal of Roe vs. Wade with the Dobbs decision has complicated this landscape further. The experiences of women who must verge on death in order to receive abortion care will ultimately result in increased maternal mortality, especially for women experiencing poverty or other barriers of access to care.

In addition to the issues of access related to politics and policy, the maternal mortality numbers for the United States reveal a deep and significant disparity in the experiences of women of color. Black and Native American women are nearly three times more likely to die in childbirth than white women in the United States. This statistic holds true across a number of other demographic factors, such as socioeconomic status and education. The root of this disparity lies in the assemblages of social factors in health that impact women of color (Trost 2023).

In the state of Georgia, reliably in the bottom tier of states for maternal mortality, there are a number of particular structural obstacles to women's healthcare. Until 2021, women who were pregnant automatically qualified for Medicaid, but coverage ended at 60 days postpartum. The data show that nearly 60 percent of maternal deaths occur in the postpartum year, so this policy effectively kept women from care when they were at their most vulnerable. It's important to note that women on Medicaid also account for 60 percent of maternal deaths (Hunter 2023). The policy was changed in July 2021 through a State Plan Amendment to include at first a six-month postpartum window as a demonstration program, and in 2023 the entire postpartum year is slated for permanent inclusion for those insured by Georgia's pregnancy Medicaid and the federal Children's Health Insurance Program

(Johnson 2023). However, at the same time, Georgia enacted a six-week abortion ban, a so-called "heartbeat" bill that prohibits abortion after six weeks. While Georgia's law is not as draconian as some, in terms of punishing doctors or patients, it still leaves most people with limited agency in their care because most people who become pregnant are not aware of the pregnancy at six weeks.

In addition to these obstacles, there are an array of social factors that intersect to have a negative impact on healthcare, in general, and on women's health in particular. Perhaps one of the most significant factors is that Georgia is predominantly rural outside of Atlanta, Savannah, Augusta, and Macon. According to data from Georgia's Rural Center, located at Abraham Baldwin Agricultural College, 26 percent of Georgians live outside urban centers and 120 of the state's 159 counties are considered rural (Georgia Rural.gov). Of Georgia's 159 counties, 56, or more than one-third, are maternity care deserts as defined by the March of Dimes. Maternity care deserts are areas with *no* obstetric facilities or services. Another 29 counties have low access to facilities or services (March of Dimes Peristats 2023). In addition, the state is experiencing a dire provider shortage. Outside of Georgia's Metropolitan Statistical Areas, there are 6.7 ob-gyns per 100,000 people, with the majority being over fifty years old (Health Georgia Data Analytics Center 2023). In addition to scarce access to healthcare providers and facilities, inequity in rural Georgia is a significant issue. People living in Georgia's rural areas experience poverty at a higher rate than urban areas (19.4 percent vs. 13 percent), with 53.8 percent having either not finished high school or earned a high school diploma as their highest level of educational attainment (U.S. Department of Agriculture Economic Research Service 2023). This compares with an 11.5 percent poverty rate for the United States overall (Shrider and Creamer 2022), and a 37 percent educational attainment rate at the high school or lower level (U.S. Census Bureau 2023). These factors combined reflect the CDC data for the country that shows that 48.9 percent of maternal mortality occurs in rural areas (Centers for Disease Control Pregnancy Mortality Surveillance System 2023).

ANTHROPOLOGY AND SYSTEMS OF CARE

In *The Birth of the Clinic* (1973), *Foucault shows us how the medical system as we know it was constructed from the observations of natural history, but codified in a new way that imbued doctors with a new and particular kind of power:*

> But the medical gaze was also organized in a new way. First, it was no longer the gaze of any observer, but that of a doctor supported and justified by an institution, that of a doctor endowed with the power of decision and intervention. Moreover, it was a gaze that was not bound by the narrow grid of structure (form, arrangement, number, size), but that could and should grasp colours, variations, tiny anomalies, always receptive to the deviant. Finally, it was a gaze that was not content to observe what was self-evident; it must make it possible to outline chances and risks; it was calculating. (89)

Foucault introduces the notion of biopower to describe how modern states exercise power over populations. Biopower operates through techniques such as regulation of birth rates, public health policies, and the management of populations. It involves not just control over individuals but also the management of life itself. His work, then, is of special interest in explorations of maternal health, and the struggle for agency in systems that control women and especially women of color.

In *Outline of a Theory of Practice* (1977), Bourdieu introduces the notion of hexis to refer to the embodied aspects of his better-known concept of habitus. Habitus, in Bourdieu's framework, is a concept that encompasses the durable and structured dispositions, habits, and inclinations that individuals develop through their socialization and experiences within a particular cultural and social context. Hexis is a visible manifestation of habitus in a person's bodily postures, gestures, and physical demeanor. Bourdieu's use of the term "hexis" refers to the embodied and often unconscious ways in which individuals physically and socially carry themselves, which are central to the themes discussed in this chapter.

Anthropologist and nurse Nancy Scheper-Hughes emphasizes that the body is not a universal biological entity but that it is culturally constructed. Her wide-ranging work has elements that touch on the data presented here, especially her work related to mothers and babies, but also her review and projections for future work in the Mindful Body (Scheper-Hughes and Lock 1987). Her work on cultural constructions of grief, infancy and motherhood (1993) are foundational to all work on these topics, including the work presented here.

Thomas Csordas is another anthropologist whose work explores the complex relationship between culture, experience, and the human body. Csordas's research (1990) emphasizes the idea that embodiment is a fundamental aspect of human existence and that it plays a central role in shaping our subjective experiences and cultural practices. Although his research focuses mainly only ritual and the cultural phenomenology practitioners and participants experience, his work is translatable to other culturally constructed and informed practices where the experiences of the body are connected to cultural practice.

In this chapter, women experiencing pregnancy go through an almost ritualistic sequence of care, in which their bodies are controlled by culturally designated specialists. From these foundations in theory, we can see the development of anthropological and other academic considerations of the pregnant body within the medical system.

Through her investigation of obstetric training in the United States, Robbie Davis-Floyd (1987) invites us to view this crucial aspect of the medical establishment as an initiatory rite of passage. All the interpretive power of symbolic anthropology is brought to bear on the sociocultural dynamics involved in the conversion of medical students into obstetricians, and we see the rites of passage, with phases of separation, transition, and integration into new social roles. Davis-Floyd takes a particular focus on the transformative liminal stage. The article emphasizes the significance of rituals and esoteric teaching in creating specialists in the medical system. Davis-Floyd discusses the emergence of humanistic birth models within obstetrics, prioritizing patient preferences, and challenging the prevailing technological birth paradigm. However, she acknowledges that these humanistic approaches face constraints imposed the authority of medical systems. The article examines how obstetricians respond to shifts in birthing practices, with younger obstetricians being more receptive to offering birthing choices but still contending with legal and financial pressures, including malpractice lawsuits. Davis-Floyd shows that the escalating use of technology and rising cesarean section rates are a consequence of the coercive influence of potential litigation.

Although young doctors find themselves caught between compassionate care and coercive legal system in Davis-Floyd's work, Monica Das Gupta (1995) emphasizes the critical role of female autonomy in shaping health outcomes for women and children. Although she compares peasant societies in preindustrial Europe and agricultural families in contemporary India, her findings are especially relevant to the discussion in this chapter because they indicate that higher autonomy is often associated with better health outcomes. The connections between autonomy, agency and outcomes is central to our examination of women's maternity care experiences in rural Georgia. Gupta also demonstrates how structural gender inequalities and societal norms limit women's autonomy, ultimately impacting their health and the health of their children.

Closer to home, Ellen Lazarus (1994) shows that women in the United States who want to exercise agency during childbirth encounter complex issues of choice and control, especially within the context social class disparities that shape women's choices. She says, "medical knowledge, like most knowledge is inseparable from social relationship and social experiences. It is unequally distributed and therefore connected to matters of power and control" (1994, 30). Further, Lazarus discusses issues of choice and control in the context of advanced medical technology, rising cesarean section rates, and the medicalization of childbirth. Ultimately, Lazarus concludes that women vary in their choices and even the awareness of their choices by social class, and she advocates for the elimination of the "two-class system of medical care to be abolished" (42). Additionally, from the data presented in this chapter that geography also plays a role in shaping women's choice, perhaps compounding Lazarus's findings.

While Lazarus is writing at the beginning of a movement to change the healthcare system—the changes proposed by the Clinton administration—she makes note of the "consumer" aspect of healthcare, in which consumers are catered to by class. By the time Christa Craven writes about "consumers" the public conversation has shifted with reproductive rights being represented as a consumer's right (2007). Craven, an anthropologist who focuses on reproductive rights, explores the "consumer identity" that is adopted in representations of reproductive healthcare and how the whole systems has felt the impact of neoliberal political shifts. In the neoliberal age, the rights and choices of self-sufficient consumers are prioritized over the human rights of citizens. Individuals who come to view themselves as healthcare consumers, must conform to the norms of the healthcare system and relinquish their broader reproductive rights. As consumers they might inadvertently lose their ability to challenge the established system and advocate for more comprehensive reproductive rights. Framing reproductive rights as consumer rights opens the way to dehumanize women participating in the healthcare system, reducing them to mere clients or commodities. In this model, healthcare providers treat patients as objects in a market-driven system rather than as unique individuals with distinct needs and rights. This dehumanization leads to control over these depersonalized bodies within healthcare, restricting women's agency and ability to shape their reproductive experiences beyond market constraints. One of the main themes in the data discussed in this chapter is the feeling of dehumanization that women experience when they engage in the medicalized birth system. In the 16 years since Craven proposed this as a model, the outcomes are readily demonstrable in women's own experiences.

The context of neoliberal capitalism is further elaborated by van der Waal et al. (2023) who emphasize the importance of understanding and addressing obstetric violence through an intersectional approach. The dehumanization and class-based system described and foretold by Lazarus and Craven are now shown to be compounded by the intersections of race, gender, location and other variables. Van der Waal et al. assert that obstetric racism is a product of historical reproductive violence and neoliberal racial capitalism. The connections between the history of obstetric violence and the health disparities that result lead van der Waal et al. to advocate for building alliances with abolitionists and social justice movements to create life-affirming medical institutions that reduce the need for obstetric intervention. They describe the abolitionist movement against obstetric violence, led by Black, Indigenous, minority, and independent midwives and doulas, and call for unity and collaboration to offer an alternative They believe that every birth has the potential to contribute to an abolitionist future by breaking down boundaries and fostering relational care (van der Waal et al. 2023).

In addition, to anthropological theories about the body and pregnant people, studies from public health, psychiatry and medical philosophy are also important to understanding our data and connect in many ways to the anthropological literature. Reaching back to the phenomenology of Csordas and his predecessors, Lewis & Holm (2023) show that knowledge of the body, and embodiment, are necessary for patients to make autonomous decisions. They emphasize the importance of understanding what they call the body's "non-cognitive, practical engagements." These are the experiences we recognize in our bodies before we reflect upon them. Our participant narratives reveal that understanding the body's intentions can contribute to a sense of empowerment. For some women, understanding "bodily intentionality" influences their ability to exercise autonomy and be involved in medical decision-making. In terms of decision-making, women also need additional information about the postpartum period and Martin et al. (2014) demonstrate that better preparation and education improve the outcomes for mothers during the postpartum period. The narratives in this chapter reflect on the postpartum experience reflect a grave need for better information and better preparation. Aside from the physical preparation women need for the postpartum period, the psychological and psychiatric needs of new mothers are often neglected in the narratives collected here. Albanese et al. (2021) show that "mothers' experiences must be central to research aimed at improving maternal postpartum mental health" (1). The data presented in this chapter reflect the need for improved maternal mental health services. In connection with these services Krapf's (2020) discussion of the need to expand the presence of doulas in the delivery room reflects the wishes of participants in this project.

THE GEORGIA MOMS PROJECT AND ITS METHODOLOGY

In 2019 author Altman had a conversation with a colleague who is an African American woman and an ob-gyn in Savannah about the emerging data that reflected Georgia's position as last for maternal mortality in the country. Although she runs a women's "safety net" clinic, serving a wide variety of women, including those experiencing poverty or lack of insurance, prior to the announcement by the CDC she had had no idea that the state numbers were so dire because in her practice they were not. Altman attended professional association meetings with her to learn about the provider side of the crisis. Most of the providers Altman encountered only knew the numbers for their own practice and many reported that they had been shocked to learn of the state's situation.

In the context of these formidable obstacles, Altman wanted to understand exactly what factors impact maternity care in Georgia from people had who had experienced it firsthand. As she and her colleague collaborated further, Altman knew that she needed to begin interviewing people about their experiences of maternity care in rural Georgia. Other studies in Georgia that have emerged focus on the clinical aspects of near misses, or postmortem interviews with the families of people who die of pregnancy-related causes. Altman wanted to understand the culture of maternity care and how women experience that culture.

Altman designed the Georgia Moms Project building on the collaboration with her colleague, and after obtaining approval from the Georgia Southern University Institutional Review Board, presented her proposal to the board of the Curtis V. Cooper Primary Health Clinics. Approval by the board would mean access to recruit patients at the clinics, and the support of the doctors and other providers on staff. Although the Georgia Moms Project had the authorization to recruit participants from social media and snowball sampling, the approval it received from the board meant that Altman could catch patients who were interested in being interviewed at her colleague's office and two other locations in Savannah. Altman also created a social media campaign to recruit participants through Facebook and a website to anonymously register particpants. The project was open to anyone who had given birth in Georgia since 2009, when the Affordable Care Act went into effect. Altman's assumption initially was that the mortality numbers must have had connections to insurance issues or access to care in rural areas. Altman constructed the interview guide around the CDC's points of potential intervention (Peterson et al. 2019) and included questions related to the patient, their family/social network, the provider, the facility where they gave birth and the healthcare system overall. Each of these points of intervention were addressed at each stage of maternity: pregnancy, labor and delivery, and the postpartum year. In addition, open-ended questions about their experiences, their feelings, and their recommendations for improving care were administered. Over forty women signed up for interviews, with thirty-eight ultimately participating, and each interview lasted an hour to ninety minutes. A demographic survey was administered before the interview and each participant was randomly assigned an ID number that they shared with me upon completion of the survey. The number was used to identify their interview and survey data to maintain their anonymity, and yet allow them a means to withdraw their data from the study if they desire. The names assigned in this chapter are pseudonyms, although the demographic data is accurate for the narrative. Each interview was transcribed using an encrypted machine transcription service, and each transcript was reviewed and corrected by student assistants. The cleaned transcripts were entered into both NVivo and Atlas-ti and coded using emergent codes with the assistance of my graduate student and coauthor Tobi Oloyede.

The demographic data reveal that about 40 percent of the participants identified as Black or mixed race, and 60 percent identified as white, and their educational and income levels varied widely. As expected, a number of cultural or social issues appeared from the coded and analyzed data, and it turned out that, of the women Altman spoke to, insurance was not a major issue, except in terms of coverage for postpartum care. One of the issues that emerged most clearly, however, is that nearly 66 percent of the interviewees reported some feeling of losing their autonomy during their maternity care experience. Twenty-five out of thirty-eight women specifically say that they were not in control of themselves during pregnancy, labor and delivery, or the postpartum year or all three. As Altman reviewed these data, new questions emerged. Do people giving birth in Georgia have a sense that they have choices in their care, and does a feeling of agency have an impact on their experience of maternity?

The narratives themselves are powerful testimony about the experience of care in the state of Georgia and the ways in which an individual can be removed from decisions that shape their own experiences and even alter their outcomes. Pregnancy can be a fraught time when pregnant people are both sharing a body with a developing human who has their own demands that sometimes override the mother's, as well as sharing (in the best case) or ceding (in many cases) control of the body to the medical establishment. Society has moved so far toward the medicalization of pregnancy that many pregnant people are unaware of their bodies' capabilities and processes at all. As soon as the pregnancy is discovered, the body of the pregnant person shifts to being a medical object, often even in their own view.

The participants have an overall awareness of their agency (or lack of agency), but their relationships with their bodies are variable. The narrative data reveal three broad themes regarding the connections between participants' experiences and their feelings of control. The three themes explored here show women experiencing an awakening of their sense of embodiment through pregnancy, the loss of agency and dehumanization they experience in mainstream medical care, and, finally, experiences of childbirth and the many complications of childbirth that can arise when decisions about the process of labor and delivery are removed from the birthing person and subsumed under the control of providers.

MATERNITY CARE NARRATIVES

When conducting the interviews, Altman asked women about their feelings of control in each of the stages of pregnancy, labor and delivery and the postpartum year. This was intended to have them reflect on their relationship with their provider and with the medical system in which they were engaged. What emerged from the data were a wide range of experiences that show that the participants rarely consider themselves in control, especially during labor and delivery. These narratives also illustrate that there can be significant consequences to women and their health outcomes when they deliver in situations where they must concede control over their bodies to medical authority.

The Body and Control

The participants who were interviewed reported various feelings of control or lack of it, but an interesting subtheme is that several of them describe their bodies as being in control, rather than themselves. This sense of complete embodiment is a fascinating aspect of pregnancy because the body controls things that we might wish otherwise in our conscious reflection and planning, especially regarding pregnancy. While planning for pregnancy, birth and the health and well-being of our children are all exercises that we engage in, we have little control over most of it. One participant, Megan (43, white) stated, "I didn't feel in control because *I felt like my body was in control. I was just like, following along.*"

In addition to being led by their bodies, other women report feelings of empowerment based on knowing their bodies and realizing that they were pregnant before testing. Alaina (33, white) says, "And then having confirmation that I was right, once we got there, and they checked on me. *That was pretty empowering. Just feeling like I could understand what my body was telling me.*" Understanding the messages of the body and knowing how to read them is an important part of developing feelings of autonomy and control. For some women, pregnancy may be their first experience of feeling this sense of embodiment or of listening to their bodies. Pregnancy becomes an urgent revelation that the experiences of their bodies are complex, mediated by culture and institutions beyond their control. With an emphasis on the body's role in autonomy, Alaina feels empowered because she can understand what her body is telling her (Lewis and Holm 2023).

Some of the participants reported strong positive feelings about pregnancy because it almost came as a surprise that most women's bodies are capable of accommodating childbirth. For some that helped them overcome some of the more difficult aspects of pregnancy and postpartum like learning to breastfeed. Anna (25, white) said that as she prepared for pregnancy she read up on other women's experiences and it helped her. She says,

> I think just reading about how other women had gone through labor and delivery and that, you know, *knowing that a woman's body is meant to do that*. I think those messages really made me feel confident, and even though I'm not like, I don't super enjoy breastfeeding, *it does make me feel really empowered because it's you know, nourishing my child with my body*.

Some of the statements about the body and childbirth indicate that pregnancy connects some women to what they see as a higher purpose or a purpose beyond what they expected, and a deeper connection to their position as mothers and women. Alex (38, white) says,

> yeah, it's crazy, but just knowing and like *the feeling that I have now, of this is what I was made to do. This is what I was meant and made to be*. Just I feel confident in that because the pregnancy was okay. The labor was okay. Like now whether I can actually . . . I have moments where I'm like, I am not adult enough to raise children. I think when I think about other people I'm like oh my god, I can't believe you have kids. You remember when we hung out at [inaudible]. Like yeah girl, I'm still that person. Like, it's weird to be like, but I am an adult, and I am responsible, and I am raising two other little people.

Pregnancy changed her view of herself and connected her to something larger. For her, motherhood is still a work in progress, expanding her ideas of her new self, but maintaining who she once knew herself to be. For some of the participants, these changing views of the self occur through the strong sense of embodiment that pregnancy demands, but it also shifts women's sense of their bodies away from the necessity to meet the demands that they express their social and cultural capital as women in society as sexually attractive or feminine (in very particular ways). Social and cultural capital expressions shift to adulthood, motherhood and all it entails.

For some participants the body was the site of self-blame and disillusionment. Jayda (42, Black) had two successful pregnancies with healthy children with her first husband. But her relationship with her second husband was exceptionally difficult, including his deployment to Afghanistan, having to quit her job that required extensive travel for the pregnancy, and a divorce before their baby's first birthday. She did not have a supportive community around her and women that she knew disapproved of her relationship and taunted her. Her body felt like the locus of all the things that were wrong, and she had a sense of foreboding throughout the pregnancy that something was amiss with her baby. When her third daughter was born, she continued to believe there was something wrong until her daughter's ultimate diagnosis with genetic disorders on her first birthday. She says,

> No, because, you know, the same body that had two other children, and is now, is now the home to a child that I don't have any control . . . I mean at the time we didn't know. But if I . . . if something was wrong, and she was inside of me, the only deduction I made was something's wrong with me. Something's wrong with her.

The connection between her body, her baby, and her feelings of guilt and shame are all deeply enmeshed. She felt out of control of the pregnancy for several reasons, but no matter how many times she tried to express her feeling that something was wrong she was never given diagnostic tests to determine whether the baby was healthy. Her knowledge of her body during pregnancy was discounted, and her concerns were attributed to her emotional state.

THE COMPLIANT BODY AND CONTROL THROUGH DEHUMANIZATION

The participants in the Georgia Moms Project were seen by ob-gyns and midwives, although the midwifery practice in the area is about an hour's drive away for many of the participants. Those who live some distance away and in the rural areas typically engage an ob-gyn. The difference in the two types of practice reflect cultural differences in the standard of care between the two types of providers, as well as the cultural backgrounds of the women who engaged midwives vs. ob-gyns. This study is small but of the fifteen women who used a midwife for at least one of their pregnancies, thirteen identified as white, one identified as Black, and one identified as "other." Invariably, the women in this study who worked with midwives reported satisfaction with their care. Women who went to both a midwife and an ob-gyn over multiple pregnancies reported glaring differences in their care. One of the most significant differences was in their feelings of dehumanization. Women attending ob-gyn appointments felt like they were engaging with a large system of care that saw them as interchangeable pieces.

Dana (39, white) reported that, "it seemed like it was control, but I really didn't have any. *I would go to the doctor, I would report, they would tell me how I was doing numbers wise, they would check something, and they would send me on my way*. That's not really control, is it?" Her only control was whether she went to the appointment or not. When she was with the provider, it didn't feel like she was actually seen. Similarly, Nelly (31, white) says, "No, I did not. Okay, why not? Um, I didn't talk. *I had no control over my pregnancy. I just, I felt almost like a robot going in that room* when I went to see the doctor and they turned me and they would tell me, okay, do this. Okay, do that. And you're just like, *okay, I'm following your direction.*" Jayda, who had difficulty delivering her third baby as described above, also felt like the care she received did not treat her as a person. She tells us, "I feel like it was just cookie cutter medicine, 'I['ve] got to see 12 million pregnant women,' and they basically just, you know, kind of herd them on through."

Jessie (44, white) felt like her visits to her providers were dehumanizing experiences as well. She describes feeling like one of many on an assembly line. She says,

> But it did really feel like I wasn't human like, *like I was on this assembly line* of like, yep, she's good. Yep, she's good, but *you didn't actually look at me*. You haven't read my chart. Because they would come in, they'd be like, which one are you? Are you the one? Did you have a C-section, and I was like, I'm *literally you delivered my baby, you know . . . Like, how, how can I pay $36,000 for a delivery and you haven't even read my chart when you're walking in here*. So, they're . . . I don't understand. I don't understand it.

We hear from her again below, where she recounts a harrowing delivery experience.

One of the most dangerous conditions associated with maternal mortality is cardiomyopathy, especially among Black women. Rhoda (40, Black) shows that one reason the condition is so deadly is that it is easy to downplay the symptoms, especially if you are busy with other children. However, she tried to tell people that she was having problems, but they assumed she was tired and out of breath because she was pregnant and caring for her other children. She says,

> With the cardiomyopathy part of it. *I think I was telling everybody there were problems*, but I think the thing is I was, what I was explaining could be just common everyday pregnancy related issues, right. So, shortness of breath. The um, um, I, I, you know, like, and I tend to downplay things because I don't like a lot of hoopla made . . . But I think when I passed out at . . . my something my children, it's one of the programs at their school or something, and *the paramedics came and then I was like, mortified*. I was like, oh my gosh, not realizing there was a problem.

Her embarrassment and desire to be an easy patient led her to further minimize the problem, and when she arrived at the hospital the interviewing nurse didn't catch the symptoms either. Rhoda continues,

> [The nurse]who was doing the evaluation sheet, you know when they were looking for fetal heartbeat, and they were like the baby sounds fine. Everything's great. Blood pressure is fine. You know? *And she said, it's probably nothing. She said, we have a nurse that works here on labor/delivery, and she passes out all the time when she's pregnant.* I'm like, okay, *so the nurse is telling me there's nothing wrong*. And *everybody's acting like it's no big deal*. Sometimes this just happens. I remember somebody saying something like the baby probably pressed your vagal nerve or something like that and. So, I was just like, well, that's what it is. But I'm, I would call [redacted] my husband and say, you know, hey, I need you to come here in a little bit, I think, because I literally feel like I'm gonna pass out. There's nothing I can do, where I can catch my breath. No matter how deeply I'm breathing. I can't catch my breath; I feel like I can't breathe. And so, he was like, well just pull over I'm coming now or whatever. *But everybody was like, that's just normal.*

She persevered through the pregnancy, but after delivering the baby, she called her ob-gyn about persistent edema in her feet and legs, and fortunately the ob-gyn listened to her other symptoms (chest pressure, shortness of breath, exhaustion, fainting) and sent her to the ER, where she was diagnosed, finally, with cardiomyopathy. For Black women, downplaying the symptoms of cardiomyopathy is one factor in it being the leading cause of pregnancy-related death.

For Joyce (39, Black) an on-call doctor changed her experience of pregnancy by revealing the sex of her babies. Her regular doctor had agreed to keep the secret, but as she tells us,

> It was around the time where I had had the Harmony test done. And my primary care doctor already knew that I didn't want to know the gender of my babies. Somewhere along [the way] the lines of communication broke down, and when he came into the room, he kind of told me and, you know, I'm pregnant. I'm almost crying, like that was, just like, I didn't . . . like it was a big deal to me. And he kind of just brushed it off, as if he was like, there's more important things to worry about, whether or not your kids are healthy and what type of twins they are. Like, he just really downplayed, like the whole thing. And it kind of, it really upset me and rubbed me the wrong way.

The shift between regular care providers that are collaborative and interested in patients as individuals, to on-call providers who have no relationship with the patient is a topic that comes up throughout the narratives from this project. Fortunately for Joyce her primary care doctor was committed to sticking with her throughout her pregnancy. When she went into the hospital to deliver her twins via C-section, her primary care provider could not perform the surgery, but he stayed in the room with her while it happened. Even with his presence in the room, she says,

> Yeah, I don't really like talking about this. *Yeah, it was my first delivery. And I had, I guess I was scared.* And I had to have the needle, the epidural. So, I was like, I don't know, like *I went into labor, like with a positive attitude when I got in that room I kind of like just got very emotional and I kind of broke down.* So, it took me a long time to, like, allow them to put the needle in and I was just emotional, and *he was just like, come on, like I could tell he would get very impatient . . . Like I didn't, he wasn't very supportive*, but mine, like I said, my doctor was in there. And he told me, he was like, you know, he was trying to encourage me, and he was saying things to me to kind of calm me down.

These narratives reflect the medicalization of the birth experience and the result of placing trust in medical diagnosis above what women are feeling, but also the disastrous provider shortage in rural Georgia. The shortage results in providers of all kinds having less and less time to spend with patients. When a patient like Joyce finds a provider that sticks with her through her C-section performed by another doctor, it is notable. When a patient like Rhoda is seen by a provider who listens and catches a hard-to-diagnose but deadly problem, it is rare.

As a point of contrast, Donna (43, white) who saw both an ob-gyn and a midwife in the Atlanta area, describes the difference in seeing a midwife compared to the ob-gyn she had also seen. She says,

> It was tremendously different. There was actually *a sense that I was a woman having a baby, not a being producing a child*, it was more about me as a person. And the baby too, but a sense that this is sort of, you know, *this is a normal, natural thing, you know, and that it wasn't alarmist, and it wasn't highly medicalized.* There was a lot less talk about numbers and percentages, but ironically, *a lot more talk about research-based care.* So, they would say, you know, the research shows x, the research shows x but, you know, we've seen x, but the research shows y, so we want to tell you about things when we decide and you helped me decide what to do about this thing.

Donna is clear that her experiences with the ob-gyn were dehumanizing visits where she was not recognized as a person. Interestingly, she also points out that her care by midwives allowed her to reflect upon the research about her choices, and that she made those choices in cooperation and collaboration with the midwives. This reflects the gulf of difference between the cultures of care available in Georgia.

The Body, Losing Control, and Obstetric Injury

Among the participants in this project, a significant number reported complications, physical injury or a lasting aftermath to their bodies following delivery. Many of these narratives feature accounts of the negotiation or challenge of control in care, and thus what emerges is that the struggle for agency is central to women's experiences of childbirth and this struggle leads to negative outcomes for some. Helena (33, white) picks up the idea that women are "meant to" have babies as mentioned by some of the narratives above. However, even though she believes that she says, "I don't like to call it breaking my body because it is what we're meant to do, and I don't think that that's conducive to my message of being pro-life, but, secretly, I don't really want to break my body again." She secretly holds her desire to keep her body safe from the difficulty of pregnancy and childbirth because she feels that conflicts with her political views. She is negotiating with herself and her position as a pro-life Christian to save her body from more damage. Most of the negotiations for care happen between the participants and their providers, but this internal conflict is of particular interest. Many Georgians, especially in rural areas, are deeply conservative, largely Christian and avowedly pro-life. This social setting puts Helena in a difficult position because she knows that after having multiple pregnancies, she does not want to be pregnant again, but she would find it difficult to refuse to carry to term if she did become pregnant.

The next three extended narratives describe the injuries that can occur to women's bodies when their autonomy is constrained or usurped by their provider. Although these narratives are explicitly about the body, there is an absolute connection to the experience of being managed by a provider, especially when the provider makes decisions based on their convenience or out of their own fear. These narratives focus on the woman's feelings upon realizing that their bodies have been injured because decisions have been made for them, often against what they had planned. In the first narrative Jessie, who complained that her provider didn't even see her above, tells of the experience of her first labor and delivery. It's a unique situation because the ob-gyn was her husband's relative, and therefore the normal boundaries between patient and provider were looser and harder to navigate. The entire family is involved in her relationship with her provider. She says,

> I was induced at 36 weeks because *he was going to Vegas, and he was our cousin and he really wanted to be there to deliver. And he was so sure because I lost my mucus plug that I was going to go into labor in the next three days,* which made the labor . . . my body was not ready. *It was an ordeal.* And so like, *I tried to go without, I wanted a natural birth. So, I'm on Pitocin and I'm trying to not get the epidural and so I felt like such a failure when like eight hours later, with Pitocin contractions, I finally said, I have to have the epidural, but I really felt like I failed.* And then he did an episiotomy so there was all that awful stuff. *He lets all the family in the room after the birth while he's stitching me up.* And I was so out of it, so, like looking back, like I hated his whole family, for like a

> year. It was really difficult, because I was like . . . my legs are in the background of some of the pictures of Granny holding the baby and I, it still makes me mad. So that's why I like, *after that episiotomy and I cannot walk, and 18 months that I couldn't have sex*, I didn't even make it to that six-week appointment. I changed to the [midwives'] birthing center because I was like *I'm going the whole radical other way than biomedicine*, give me a witch doctor, or whatever, you know what I mean. *Whatever, just not that*. yeah, I literally went like, I've never thought about a midwife in my life, but we're gonna find one.

Throughout the beginning of her narrative, we can see that most of the arrangements for her first labor and delivery experience are being made to accommodate the doctor who is her husband's cousin. Her labor was induced against her original wishes for a natural vaginal delivery, and because she couldn't have the natural birth she had planned, she feels like a failure for having an epidural. She internalizes the blame for choices that she was unable to make because the doctor asserted control over her experience. Further, he takes control of the post birth moment and allows the extended family into the delivery room while she is still being treated. Her anger was palpable in this interview even though this child was a teenager at the time of the interview. The physical effects of the episiotomy left her with pain and difficulty for a year and a half. The experience changed her perspective not only of herself, but of the family and the biomedical approach to pregnancy.

The next narrative, provided by Courtney (32, Black and white) is made even more disheartening when we realize that she works in the health professions in an OB-GYN office. She had had one successful pregnancy, but during her second pregnancy the baby was quite large and presented potential problems with delivery. She, with her professional knowledge, and her doula had discussed the potential problems, and had a plan for delivering naturally, if possible. In this particular delivery her regular doctor was not on call, and she went into delivery to find that she was being cared for by a stranger, who she said was, "brand new. I [could] see the peach fuzz like on his chin. He's new new. He just got out of med school." However, she and her husband had a plan and a supportive doula who was there to advocate for her as she labored and began to deliver. She tells us,

> [The doula says] You are good at this. You did a great job your first time. You can do it the second time. And she said she kept giving me, like, positive affirmations. Like, your body's not going to make a baby you can't push out you, you know this, just keeping me cool, calm and collected. *I wanted to push slowly because I didn't want to have another third-degree tear.* So, I did, I pushed slowly, *I listened to my body*. I got her head out. And when I got her head out, I didn't have another contraction. *And everyone freaked out*. They called a code dystocia, *another doctor came in, another doctor came in, two more nurses*

came in. They dropped me completely flat on my back. And I was like, um, I can't push like this. I need someone to help me sit up and I looked around. *My husband and my doula are gone. I'm just surrounded by medical staff now. And I'm like, I need help.* And I'm trying to sit up on my own and I just can't do it. And they're like you need to push right now you need to push. And I was like, I'm not having a contraction, can we wait for the next contraction. *And, so, the nurse just applied fundal pressure*, and was like, we need to get this baby out now. And then the baby was out. *Right before she completely left my body. I felt a searing pain in my perineum.* [They called] a shoulder dystocia but they called it really quickly. And I thought that was weird because usually it takes like, at least two minutes for them to call it and by the operative (I got my operative notes or like the whatever notes afterwards) and they were weird too. *They said that a code shoulder dystocia was called, but there was no shoulder dystocia.* But a neonatologist came and talked to me about potential physical therapy for her shoulder. So, I don't know . . .

Interviewer: So, once she was born, did she have problems with her shoulder?

Speaker 2: She was fine. The only thing that was weird looking about her is that she was 11 pounds. So, she was huge. And she had really bad Tiki eye [petechial hemorrhage]. So, all the whites in her eyes were completely red, so I knew that there was a lot of cranial pressure. *So, I knew that that was why he was freaking out. He needed her to come out, I get it. None of that, I guess was really communicated to me because I wasn't, I was trying to do it slowly* . . . But *he did give me an episiotomy, right on top of my tear*. And then *he took about five seconds to sew it back up*. And it took forever to heal. And when I didn't, well, right immediately afterwards, I just kind of sat there and stared up at the ceiling forever and I was incredibly cold. And I was just like, where is everybody? And um, it was just *I don't know how long I was flat on my back with people on me. But that feeling of like, helplessness and the loss of autonomy messed me up really bad.* And I ended up having to like, seek counseling to talk about it. But even when I talked to my doctor, I was like, I feel like I'm not healing up properly. Like it just it feels differently. And *he was like, well, you know, you had an 11-pound baby. Ha ha,* you know. And I'm like, Okay, cool. I switched doctors, and *I said that I felt like I almost had PTSD* after having this delivery experience. And *she was like, well, you did have an 11-pound baby*. I see why, but no *one ever referred me to any psychiatric help*. And so, I talked to my doula friend about it, and she recommended somebody, but I really feel like my healthcare providers shouldn't have been like . . . she's making PTSD jokes.

This was a very difficult interview because she was still having complicated feelings about her birth experience and there was so much that had gone wrong. Her episiotomy was not repaired properly, she experienced an extended period of edema and water retention after leaving the hospital, and even at the time of the interview (four years later) she was still experiencing issues with her pelvic floor. In this particular case, instead of the doctor overriding the patient's preferences for his own convenience, the provider is afraid or perhaps risk-averse and uncommunicative. Instead of the slow, deliberate, calm birth she had planned, her doula was pushed aside, the doctor called for an emergency team, and she was physically held down and the baby pushed out of her body. This is an actual lifesaving maneuver if the birth is obstructed, but it is not clear that that is what happened, at least not to Courtney. Instead, she was treated as a medical object and kept in the dark about what was happening and why. When the authority over our bodies is vested in the medical system, we enter into a trust relationship with the providers who are supposed to care for us. In delivery rooms, where the medical authority rotates to whomever is on call, our trust must then be assigned to the system that trains, regulates and assigns the providers who have control. We must trust that their knowledge, their tolerance for risk, and their ability to communicate will provide a labor and delivery that aligns with our expectations. Courtney laments the loss of her autonomy, a loss that has caused her continuing mental health issues as well as damage to her body. For her, one of the most critical moments of her life was under the control of someone she did not know, someone who was not communicative and someone who, from her perspective, panicked when things did not go as he expected. Beyond the immediate experience of labor and delivery, Courtney also had two different doctors make light of her asking for help with what she considered to be PTSD. Having a large baby, alone, is not necessarily a traumatic experience. The interventions of the medical staff left her with feelings of having been violated, not the experience of having a large baby.

In Courtney's narrative, the doula provides emotional support and encouragement during childbirth, aligning with Krapf's (2020) description of the role of doulas in the birthing process. She discusses how doulas offer continuous physical, emotional, and informational support to mothers during childbirth. Courtney described how she felt pressured to push quickly, which echoes Krapf's discussion of the medicalization of birth and how doulas often find themselves in the role of supporting individuals within the medicalized hospital system. Krapf raises questions about the limitations of doulas in challenging the systemic issues within the medicalized birth system. In this context, Courtney's experience illustrates the challenges faced by individuals during childbirth and highlights the need for advocates like doulas who can support birthing individuals in asserting their preferences and rights within the healthcare system. Krapf (2020) depicts the doula's role as a potential change agent within the medical institution and the limitations they may encounter in advocating for more holistic and patient-centered birthing experiences. Georgia piloted Medicaid support for doulas, with that pilot phase ending in 2023 (Healthy Mothers Healthy Babies of Georgia 2023).

Further, Courtney's feeling of being ignored by healthcare providers illustrates the disconnect between what postpartum women perceive as their concerns and what healthcare providers prioritize (Martin et al. 2014). In addition, Albanese et al. (2021) discuss the gap between what mothers want from postpartum care and what is actually offered. They underscore the neglect of the maternal psychosocial experience in postpartum care, where mothers often feel unprepared, overwhelmed, and unsupported due to inadequate care, which can lead to negative mental health consequences. It emphasizes the importance of patient-centered care and involvement in decision-making, highlighting the need for a shift towards more patient-centered protocols.

As dramatic as Jessie and Courtney's labor and delivery experiences were, participants also reported long-lasting physical injury that occurred during labor and delivery, but which did not become apparent until later. For Megan (43, white) this took the form of a rectocele (a form of vaginal prolapse) that she lived with for months, because she didn't know that it was not normal, and was trying to figure it out on her own. Her narrative is filled with hedges and hesitations because she still found this difficult to talk about.

> But mostly, like, I worried about . . . so after my first one, so I ripped with both. So, I had to get stitched up. So, like, that's painful. And, um, my first one like, I was already *like having pain when I was having a bowel movement*. So, I wasn't sure if that was normal. *But it was searing pain*. It was like *that was scary cause I was like, I don't even know what was happening*. Like, I don't know why. I don't know if that's like the stitches or what, um, and then maybe like *a couple years after*, I don't even know when this occurred, definitely before my second pregnancy, I developed a rectocele. So, I had no idea this could happen. Like I had no idea. *Like your body can end up being basically ruined by having a baby*. So, so then I was thinking maybe that's what that searing pain was like, my actual, like tissues kind of like, ripping or I don't know, just like the integrity of the tissues, just like we're done. And so, I guess like, *I worried about my body being able to work properly, you know, like basically, having your vagina be done, you know, like, no elasticity*. Everything's just blown out and is trying to fall out. Like, that is like . . . *that's something I didn't realize could happen*. And then when it did, I was like, oh, well, okay, *so then how does this ever get fixed like, what do I plan for now*?

Megan struggled with pain and difficult bowel movements for nearly two years before asking her provider about the rectocele, and then felt that her body had been ruined forever. While a rectocele results from thinned or damaged perineal tissue and is difficult to prevent from happening during delivery or postpartum, she received no education that this could be a potential problem. Early intervention is important to make repair or treatment more effective, and pelvic floor strengthening exercises before or after delivery can mitigate the problem. While this information is readily available through medical websites that allow self-diagnosis, her shame, fear and confusion kept her from asking her provider until it became a significant issue as she was considering a second pregnancy. The surprise that changes in the body after pregnancy can be lifelong and substantial could also be mitigated by better communication and education. Megan's experience reflects several key themes discussed in Martin et al. (2014), including the lack of knowledge and preparation many women have regarding postpartum health. The obvious need for better communication and support aligns with recommendations by Martin et al. (2014) for improving postpartum care.

DISCUSSION AND CONCLUSIONS

The narratives collected as part of the Georgia Moms Project form a corpus that allow us to examine a broad cross section of questions through a few different lenses. We can see in the narratives selected here echoes of Foucault's positions on biopower, governmentality, the body politic and centralization of knowledge. We can see Bourdieu's model of the body as hexis, where the cultural and social practices are manifest. We can see the embodiment of culture as women experiences, and the cultural construction of the bodies that are described here.

The themes reflected in the data indicate that the participants largely do not feel a sense of embodiment until their pregnancy makes it unavoidable. They are pulled into feeling the new and challenging experiences of their bodies with varying results. For some, a positive connection to the larger world, for some a sense of loss of control. Further, when women seek care for their pregnancy, they often feel dehumanized. The medical establishment as it currently exists leaves little time for meaningful interaction with their providers and they feel as though they are just one of many, as well as feeling frightened or ashamed to ask questions. Finally, when women are fully engaged in the birthing process, they lose all control of their bodies, and when hurried, inexperienced, or unfamiliar providers take over, injury can result. It is not acceptable for the obstetric injuries that occurred to these women to be the result of convenience, risk aversion or failure to communicate.

Whether we view these women's experiences as a reflection of the neoliberal policies that have shifted medical care to a model that prioritizes the health of institutions over the health of individual patients and the individual practices of providers, or we see the bodies of these women as the locus for control between themselves and the medical establishment, the outcomes are the same. Women are dying at an alarming rate in the state of Georgia, and the women who survive their maternity experience and recount their experiences often have lasting feelings of dehumanization and in some cases lasting damage to both their bodies and psyches. The women who have a better understanding of the work their bodies can do show us that if women are encouraged to develop a sense of empowerment and afforded a level of autonomy, they can experience that power in ways that aid their labor, delivery, and recovery. Women who are overruled without communication from their providers or who have their agency usurped by providers struggle not only with their experiences of labor and delivery, but with their mental health after delivery and sometimes for years after.

If we were to propose solutions to the issues revealed by these narratives, we would echo the findings of work being done across the country. First, the provider shorter in Georgia must be addressed. More providers, especially in rural areas, would mean more time spent per patient and the development of closer relationships. Closer relationships between providers and patients would facilitate better communication throughout pregnancy and crucially during labor and delivery and during the postpartum year. The medical establishment must shift to a model of patient-centered care that features this type of relationship building and communication as a hallmark. Additionally, the inclusion of supportive care in the form of doulas during all phases of maternity would better connect the patient to the processes taking place in their own bodies and connect them to cultural practices that have been obscured by the models of medicalization that dominate the landscape of maternity care. The expansion of roles (including improved reimbursement policies through Medicaid and employer-sponsored insurance) for midwives, doulas, and other specialists in patient centered birth care could alleviate both the provider shortage and the need to develop closer connections. Finally, women of all ages need better education about their bodies, about what their bodies are experiencing and how they can exercise agency over their health, well-being, and interactions with the medical establishment.

REFERENCES CITED

Albanese, Ariana M., Pamela A. Geller, Christina A. Sikes, and Jennifer L. Barkin. 2021. "The Importance of Patient-Centered Research in the Promotion of Postpartum Mental Health." *Frontiers in Psychiatry* 12.

Bourdieu, Pierre. 1977. *Outline of a Theory of Practice*. Translated by Richard Nice. Cambridge: Cambridge University Press.

Craven, Christa. 2007. "A 'Consumer's Right' to Choose a Midwife: Shifting Meanings for Reproductive Rights under Neoliberalism." *American Anthropologist* 109 (4): 701–12.

Csordas, Thomas J. 1990. "Embodiment as a Paradigm for Anthropology." *Ethos* 18 (1): 5–47.

Davis-Floyd, Robbie E. 1987. "Obstetric Training As a Rite of Passage." *Medical Anthropology Quarterly* 1 (3): 288–318.

Doepke, Matthias, Michèle Tertilt, and Alessandra Voena. 2012. "The Economics and Politics of Women's Rights." *Annual Review of Economics* 4: 339–72.

"Doula Medicaid Reimbursement Pilot." n.d. Healthy Mothers, Healthy Babies Coalition of Georgia. Accessed October 8, 2023. https://www.hmhbga.org/advocacy/doula-medicaid-reimbursement-pilot.

Foucault, Michel. 1973. *The Birth of the Clinic: An Archaeology of Medical Perception*. Translated by A. M. Sheridan. London: Routledge.

"Georgia | RURAL.Gov." 2023. February 1, 2023. Accessed October 8, 2023. https://www.rural.gov/community-networks/ga.

Gupta, M. D. 1995. "Life Course Perspectives on Women's Autonomy and Health Outcomes." *American Anthropologist*, 97 (3), 481–91.

"Health | Georgia Data Analytics Center." n.d. Accessed October 7, 2023. https://gdac.georgia.gov/health-0.

Hunter, Kenya. 2023. "The Biggest Barrier to State-Funded Doulas for Pregnant Women." Capital B Atlanta. August 21, 2023. Accessed August 8, 2023. https://atlanta.capitalbnews.org/maternal-health-doula-legislation/.

Johnson, Maureen. 2023. "Georgia Extends Medicaid Postpartum Coverage for Pregnant Women." *NASHP* (blog). April 24, 2023. Accessed August 8, 2023. https://nashp.org/georgia-extends-medicaid-postpartum-coverage-for-pregnant-women/.

Krapf, Jasmine. 2020. "Addressing the Doula Paradox: An Analysis and Reimagining of a Changing Role in Reproductive Justice." *Student Anthropologist* 7 (1): 29–41.

Lazarus, Ellen S. 1994. "What Do Women Want?: Issues of Choice, Control, and Class in Pregnancy and Childbirth." *Medical Anthropology Quarterly* 8 (1): 25–46.

Lewis, Jonathan, and Søren Holm. 2023. "Towards a Concept of Embodied Autonomy: In What Ways Can a Patient's Body Contribute to the Autonomy of Medical Decisions?" *Medicine, Health Care and Philosophy*, June.

Martin, Anika, Carol Horowitz, Amy Balbierz, and Elizabeth Howell. 2014. "Views of Women and Clinicians on Postpartum Preparation and Recovery." *Maternal & Child Health Journal* 18 (3): 707–13.

"Peristats | March of Dimes." n.d. March of Dimes | PeriStats. Accessed October 7, 2023. https://www.marchofdimes.org/peristats/.

Petersen, Emily E., Nicole L. Davis, David Goodman, Shanna Cox, Nikki Mayes, Emily Johnston, Carla Syverson et al. 2019. "Vital Signs: Pregnancy-Related Deaths, United States, 2011–2015, and Strategies for Prevention, 13 States, 2013–2017." *MMWR. Morbidity and Mortality Weekly Report* 68 (18): 423–29.

"Pregnancy Mortality Surveillance System | Maternal and Infant Health | CDC." March 31, 2023. Center for Disease Control and Prevention. Accessed October 8, 2023. https://www.cdc.gov/reproductivehealth/maternal-mortality/pregnancy-mortality-surveillance-system.htm.

Reyes-Foster, Beatriz M. 2023. "'No Justice in Birth': Maternal Vanishing, VBAC, and Reconstitutive Practice in Central Florida." *American Anthropologist* 125 (1): 49–62.

Scheper-Hughes, Nancy. 1993. *Death Without Weeping: The Violence of Everyday Life in Brazil*. Berkeley: University of California Press.

Scheper-Hughes, Nancy, and Margaret M. Lock. 1987. "The Mindful Body: A Prolegomenon to Future Work in Medical Anthropology." *Medical Anthropology Quarterly* 1 (1): 6–41.

Shrider, Emily A, and John Creamer. 2023. US Census Bureau, "Poverty in the United States: 2022." Accessed October 8, 2023. https://www.census.gov/content/dam/Census/library/publications/2023/demo/p60-280.pdf.

Tikkanen, Roosa, Munira Z. Gunja, Molly FitzGerald, and Laurie C. Zephyrin. November 18, 2020 "Maternal Mortality and Maternity Care in the United States Compared to 10 Other Developed Countries." 2020. The Commonwealth Fund Website. Accessed August 8, 2023. https://www.commonwealthfund.org/publications/issue-briefs/2020/nov/maternal-mortality-maternity-care-us-compared-10-countries.

Trost, Susanna, Jennifer Beauregard, Gyan Chandra, Fanny Njie, Jasmine Berry, and David A Goodman. n.d. "Pregnancy-Related Deaths: Data from Maternal Mortality Review Committees in 36 US States, 2017–2019," 6.

U.S. Census Bureau. n.d. "Educational Attainment in the United States: 2022." Census.Gov. Accessed October 7, 2023. https://www.census.gov/data/tables/2022/demo/educational-attainment/cps-detailed-tables.html.

U.S. Department of Agriculture. 2023. "State Data." August 31, 2023. US Department of Agriculture, Economic Research Service. Accessed October 8, 2023. https://data.ers.usda.gov/reports.aspx?StateFIPS=13&StateName=Georgia&ID=17854.

Valencia, Zehra, Aditi Sen, Debra Bozzi, Katie Martin, and Daniel Kurowski. n.d. "One-Third of Births Occurred by C-Section in ESI and Medicaid in 2020." HCCI. Accessed October 8, 2023. https://healthcostinstitute.org/hcci-originals-dropdown/all-hcci-reports/one-third-of-births-occurred-by-c-section-in-esi-and-medicaid-in-2020-1

Waal, Rodante van der, Kaveri Mayra, Anna Horn, and Rachelle Chadwick. 2023. "Obstetric Violence: An Intersectional Refraction through Abolition Feminism." *Feminist Anthropology* 4 (1): 91–114.

Index

About the Contributors

Dorcas Ama Adom is a graduate student in Community health at the Jiann Ping Hsu College of Public Health, Georgia Southern University. She holds a bachelor's degree in physician assistantship from Presbyterian University Ghana. Dorcas is a certified physician assistant with over two years' clinical management and community engagement. In her current studies, Dorcas engages in research that is centered on health equity and health disparities. She is a graduate assistant at the Office of Health Equity and Community Engagement, where she facilitates and assists in creating spaces for community engagement with research findings to inform new community-led initiatives. She is particularly interested in HIV/AIDS prevention, substance use management and rehabilitation, and community engagement. Adom is expected to graduate in May 2024, and she is exploring PhD positions in behavioral and social sciences and public health informatics.

Heidi M. Altman, PhD, is an applied anthropologist who has worked in Native American and African American communities in North Carolina, Oklahoma, California, Mexico, Canada, New York, Georgia, and elsewhere, to help identify and resolve issues being experienced in those communities. Much of this work has been done as a consultant or in conjunction with nonprofit work, and includes a problem gambling assessment, language revitalization initiatives, an exploration of the reestablishment of traditional midwifery practices, behavioral health projects related to diabetes prevention, the expansion of public Wi-Fi during the pandemic, and the development of after-school programs for underserved children. All of these projects have been built around community input (community-based participatory research) and therefore are centered on interviews, focus groups, surveys and other methods of gathering information about community needs and issues. In order to access these communities, she has committed years of effort to building relationships, social networks, and trust. Altman has a current research project underway that seeks to understand how mothers experience the maternal health crisis in Georgia by interviewing women about their lived experience of maternity care. This research has taken a special focus on the disparities experienced by African American women who are affected by maternal mortality at a rate three to five times higher than their white counterparts in Georgia.

Jacqueline Berger, PhD, is an applied biological anthropologist at Georgia Southern University who has conducted anthropological research in the Southeastern United States (Georgia, Florida, Mississippi, and Texas), the Western United States (California, Colorado, Montana, and Wyoming), and Italy. While completing a PhD in applied anthropology at University of South Florida (2021), she also served as the associate director of research programs for the Center for Health Equity, Education, and Research at Boston Medical Center. Her research investigates the historical anatomization of institutionalized individuals, especially skeletal trauma and taphonomy in these populations, combining bioarchaeological and forensic anthropological methods and theory.

Bryan Fluech is the associate Marine Extension director for University of Georgia Marine Extension and Georgia Sea Grant. Fluech is a trained science educator, with extensive experience in outreach and extension work. He has been working across the South Atlantic region for over fifteen years.

Anne O. Odusanya, Dr. PH., MPH, has a decade of public health experience, specifically related to maternal and child health (MCH) regarding community health behavior and education. This includes creating undergraduate and graduate curricula, working alongside minoritized communities (BIPOC, LGBTQIA+, and families of children and youth with special health care needs [CYSHCN]), in addition to equity-oriented program development, implementation, and evaluation nationally and internationally.

Tobi Oloyede is a public health doctoral student at Georgia Southern University (GSU). She holds a master of social science (sociology) degree from GSU and another master of arts in liberal studies (gender and diversity) degree from East Tennessee State University. She completed her undergraduate degree in Nigeria, where she graduated with a bachelor of arts in English and literary studies from Ekiti State University. Tobi's research revolves around maternal and child health, social determinants of health, and health equity. She leverages human-centered design (HCD) techniques to understand and address individual, business, and community needs.

Stacy W. Smallwood, PhD, is an associate professor of community health behavior and education at the Jiann-Ping Hsu College of Public Health at Georgia Southern University. He has more than twenty years of experience with community-engaged approaches to health promotion, including the use of multi-method and mixed-method research designs. He also has extensive experience in public health capacity-building and leadership development. From 2004 to 2010, he served in diverse management and leadership roles within the CDC/ASPH Institute for HIV Prevention Leadership (IHPL), an intensive capacity-building program for HIV prevention program managers from community-based organizations across the United States and its territories.

Cindi SturtzSreetharan, PhD, received her PhD in linguistic anthropology from UC Davis. She is an associate professor in the School of Human Evolution and Social Change at Arizona State University. As a current Abe Fellow, SturtzSreetharan has been working at the intersection of masculinity, obesity, and stigma in both US and Japan contexts. Her recent cross-cultural ethnography, *Fat in Four Cultures* (University of Texas Press), examines the lived experience of women and weight in Japan, Samoa, Paraguay, and the United States. Her current project aims to learn more about how men's lives are impacted by their experiences of fat and overweight. She is particularly interested in the role that health policy plays in felt stigma around body size.

Jennifer Sweeney Tookes, PhD, is an applied cultural anthropologist at Georgia Southern University who has conducted anthropological research in the Southeastern United States (Georgia and South Carolina) and the Caribbean (Barbados, US Virgin Islands) since 2003. After completing a PhD in anthropology at Emory University (2013), her postdoctoral training in environmental sciences (2014–2016) investigated the potential for Georgia seafood producers to participate in active local foods movements. Her research bridges medical and environmental anthropology, focusing on changing sea levels and climate, seafood production, coastal communities, and the health, well-being, and cultural heritage of these populations. Tookes is the vice chair of the SocioEconomic Panel of the South Atlantic Fishery Management Council (SAFMC), and serves on the Science and Statistics Committee for the council. She is active in the Society for Applied Anthropology.

Cassandra White, PhD, (she/her/hers) is an associate professor in the department of anthropology at Georgia State. She is a cultural and medical anthropologist who focuses on Latin America and the United States in her research. She directed seven anthropology field schools in Brazil between 2005 and 2018. The complex and intersecting factors involved in the construction of stigma and the subsequent discrimination and exclusion that can result from that stigma have been themes that connect a diverse set of research projects and interests. Much of her research over the past twenty-five years has focused on experiences of people affected by Hansen's disease (leprosy) in Brazil and the United States. Her book *An Uncertain Cure: Living with Leprosy in Rio de Janeiro* (Rutgers University Press, 2009) is based on this research. She has also conducted research on immigration and health in the Atlanta metropolitan area, racial identity among Brazilian Americans in Atlanta, spirit mediumship in the United States and Brazil, the effects of mega-events on residents of Rio de Janeiro, and experiences of extended breastfeeding/chestfeeding in the United States.

Tracy Yandle was an Associate Professor of Environmental Science at Emory University for twenty years. She completed her PhD in public policy at Indiana University Bloomington studying natural resource management with Nobel Prize–winning scholar Elinor Ostrom. During her time at Emory, her research focused on fishers' interactions with institutions and social and economic incentives. She also served multiple terms on the South Atlantic Fishery Council's Scientific and Statistical Committee and Social-Economic Panel. She is now a senior adviser at the New Zealand Ministry of Transport.

www.ingramcontent.com/pod-product-compliance
Ingram Content Group UK Ltd.
Pitfield, Milton Keynes, MK11 3LW, UK
UKHW041838031026
15587UKWH00002B/851

9 781666 952704